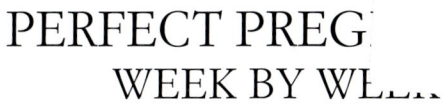

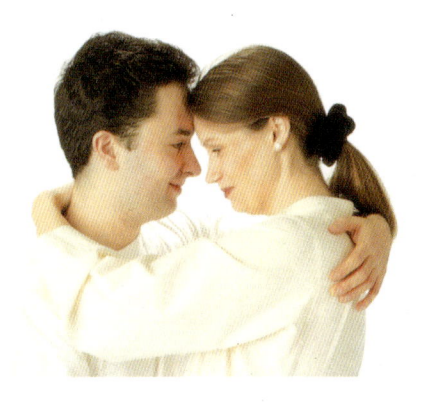

PRACTICAL HAN

PERFECT PREG
WEEK BY WEEK

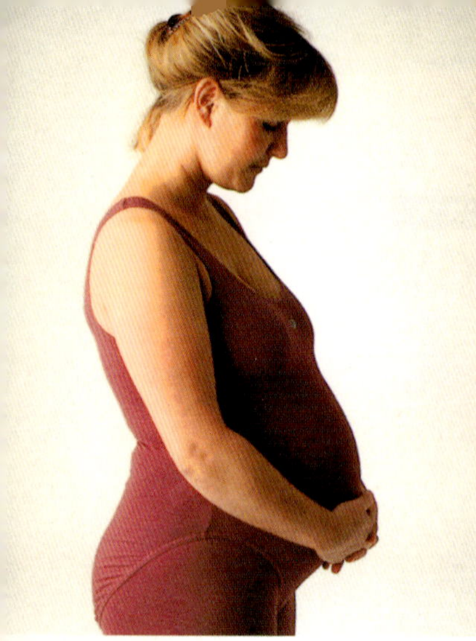
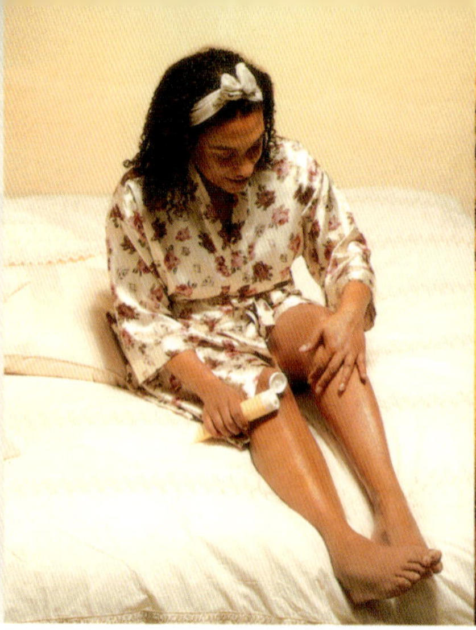
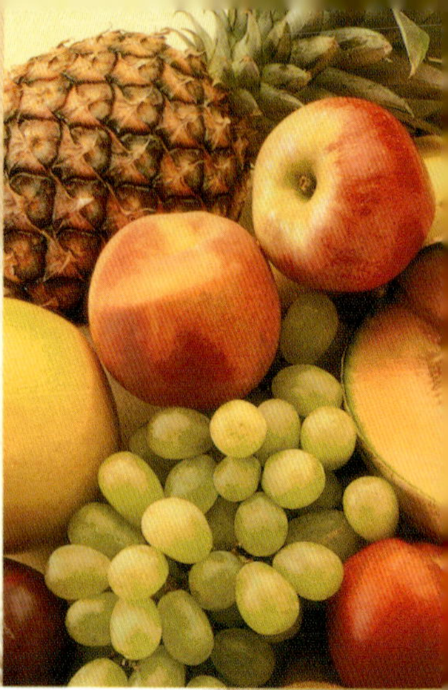
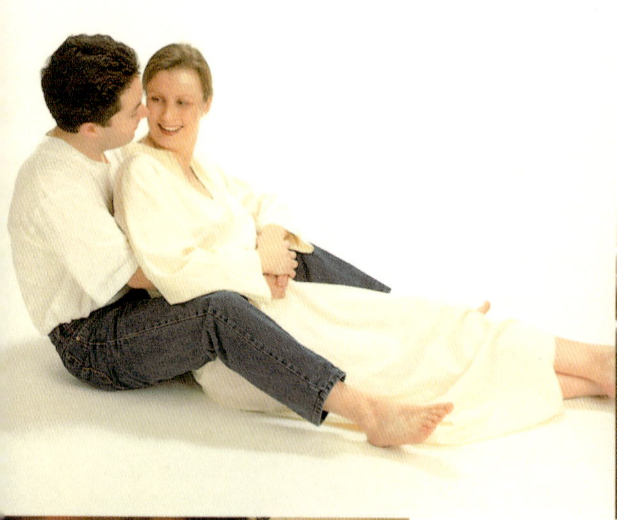
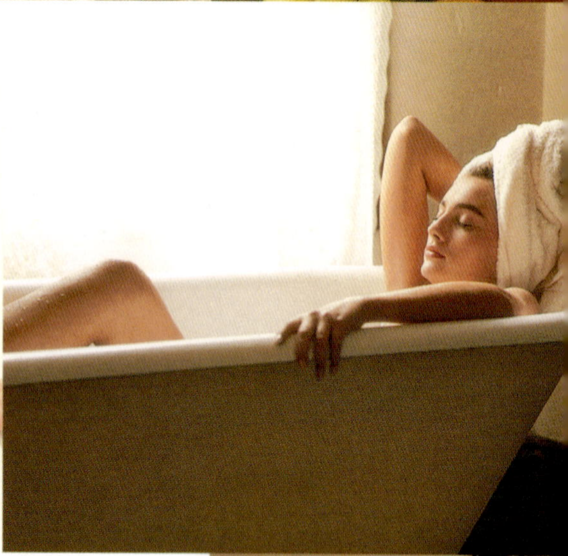
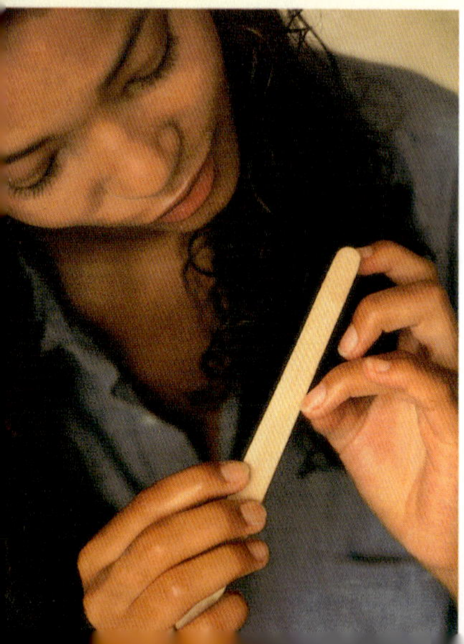
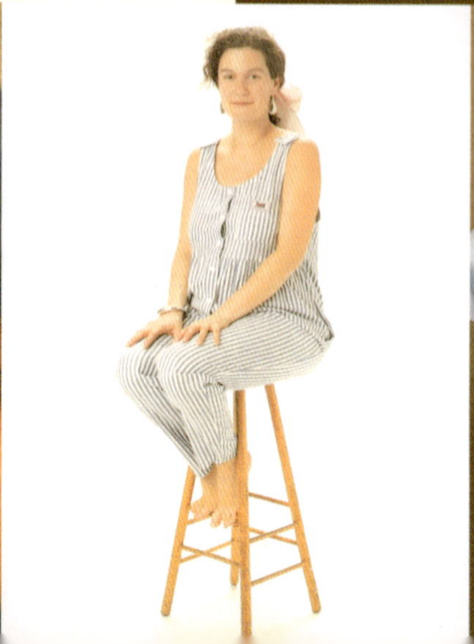
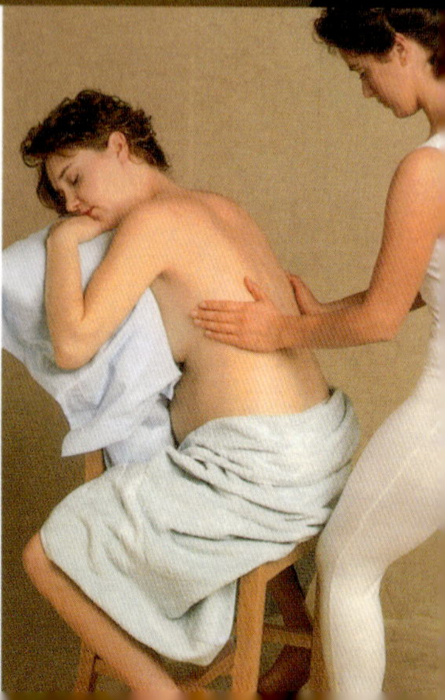

PRACTICAL HANDBOOK

PERFECT PREGNANCY
WEEK BY WEEK

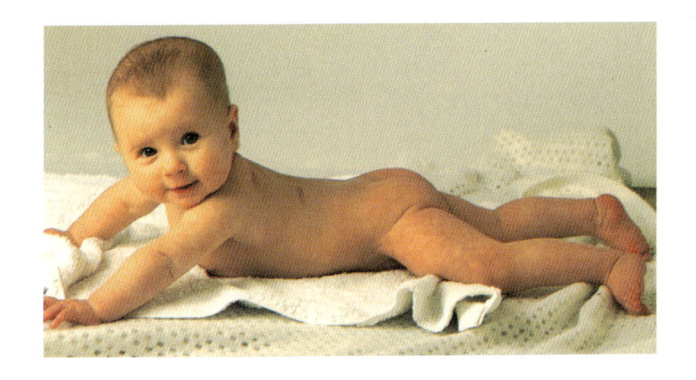

ALISON MACKONOCHIE

Sebastian Kelly

A VERY SPECIAL THANK YOU TO ROBIN FOR HIS UNFAILING SUPPORT, TO LUCY AND KATE, WITHOUT WHOM WE WOULD NOT HAVE HAD CHRISTMAS, AND TO DOMINIC FOR JUST BEING HIMSELF.

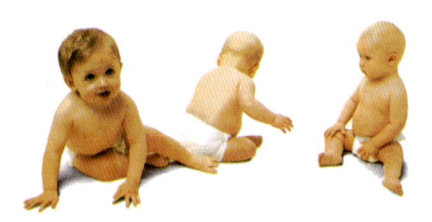

This edition published by
Sebastian Kelly
2 Rectory Road, Oxford OX4 1BW

© Anness Publishing Limited 1996, 1999

Produced by
Anness Publishing Limited
Hermes House
88-89 Blackfriars Road
London SE1 8HA

All rights reserved. No part of this publication may be reproduced, stored in a retrieval system, or transmitted in any way or by any means, electronic, mechanical, photocopying, recording or otherwise, without the prior written permission of the copyright holder.

A CIP catalogue record for this book is available from the British Library

ISBN 1-84081-236-2

Also published as *Your Pregnancy Week by Week*, and as part of a larger compendium, *The Complete Book of Pregnancy & Babycare*.

Publisher: Joanna Lorenz
Project Editors: Casey Horton, Nicky Thompson
Editor: Elizabeth Longley
Designer: Bobbie Colgate-Stone
Special Photography: Alistair Hughes
Additional Photography: Carin Simon
Illustrations: Ian Sidaway
Hair and Make-up: Bettina Graham
Cover Design: Balley Design Associates

Printed and bound in Hong Kong

10 9 8 7 6 5 4 3 2 1

ACKNOWLEDGEMENTS
The author and publisher would like to thank the many individuals who helped in the creation of this book. Particular thanks are due to Bobbie Brown, Elsa Jacobi, Pauline Richardson, Mary Lambert and Jane Barret. Many thanks also go to everyone who modelled for special photography: Yvonne Adams and Martin; Ruth Auber and Bethany; Jo Bates and Lois; Amanda Bennet-Jones; Kim, Neil and Andrew Brown; Christine Clarke; Jacqueline Clarke and Cassia; Jocelyn Cusack and Beth; Sam Dyas and Colt; Patricia Gannon and Matthew; Nici Giles and Fergus; Yiota Gillis and Cameron; Sandra Hadfield and Annie; Louise Henriques and Joshua; Lynette Jones and Hugh and Rhys; Karen, Mark, Megan and Robert Lambert; Claire Lehain and Harriet; Lavinia Mainds and Polly; Pippa Milton and Oliver; Philippa Madden and Inca; Jackie Norbury; Jess Presland; Katey Steiner; Saatchi Spracklen and Niamh; Sophie Trotter and Archie; Josephine Whitfield and Lily May; Lucinda Whitrow and Hector. Thanks also to companies who loaned items and photographs: Blooming Marvellous Ltd (pages 36-37), Boots Children's Wear and Toys, Fisher-Price, Littlewoods Home Shopping, Maclaren Ltd and Mattel UK Ltd.

Picture acknowledgements: **Bubbles** 74; /Jacquie Farrow, 64, /Julie Fisher 5, /Nikki Gibbs 12 b, 76; /Paul Howard 71 t; /Julia Martin 17 b, 81 (all 3); /Loisjoy Thurston 1, 25 b, 43 t and r 48, 60, 77; /Ian West 73 b; /J. Woodcock 25 t, 74; /Richard Yard 65; **Lupe Cunha** 14, 15, 17 t and b, 19, 22, 23 b, 29 t and b, 35 t, 48, 49 t, 57 bl and t, 57 r, 69 t, 78, 82, 83; **PR Communications** 50 (box); **Science Photo Library**/BSIP Bajande 85 b; /Mark Clarke 56, 57 t, 68, 69 b, 70, 71 b, 75 r, 84 t and b, 85 t and b; /Custom Medical Stock 57 t, 85 t; /Simon Fraser 43, 69 b; /Will & Deni McIntyre 20 t, 21 b; /Joseph Mettis 68; /Petit Format/Nestle 12 t; /Chris Priest 32; 35; /Richard G Rawlins 11 tl, 20 t, 21 b, 31, 32; /Pascale Roche/Petit Format 84 t and b; /James Stevenson 16 br, 31 b, 43 bl; /Ron Sutherland 75 r; /Sheila Terry 17 t, 61, 79 bl; /Jonathan Watts 56; **Carin Simon** 76 r.
(**Key**: b – bottom, bl – bottom left, br – bottom right, r – right, t – top, tl – top left, tr – top right).

CONTENTS

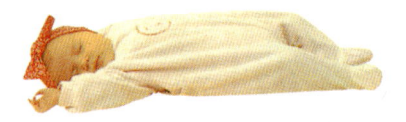

INTRODUCTION 6

Preparing For Pregnancy 8
THE FIRST TRIMESTER
Weeks 1-4: Conception 10 • Week 5: Confirming Pregnancy 12 • Week 6: Ante-natal Choices 14 • Week 7: Possible Problems 16 • Week 8: Booking-in/Routine Tests 18 • Week 9: Special Tests 20 • Week 10: Hormones/Maternity Record 22 • Week 11: Common Discomforts 24 • Week 12: Healthy Eating 26 • Week 13: The Health Professionals 28
THE SECOND TRIMESTER
Week 14: Sex During Pregnancy 30 • Week 15: Health and Safety 32 • Week 16: Scans/Twins 34 • Week 17: Your Pregnancy Wardrobe 36 • Week 18: Looking Your Best 38 • Week 19: Exercise 40 • Week 20: Skin Care/Cravings 42 • Week 21: Minor Complaints 44 • Week 22: Relaxation and Massage 46 • Week 23: Preparing the Nursery 48 • Week 24: Baby Clothes and Equipment 50 • Week 25: Feeding Choices 52 • Week 26: Parentcraft Classes 54
THE THIRD TRIMESTER
Week 27: Choices in Childbirth 56 • Week 28: The Birthplan 58 • Week 29: Special Care 60 • Week 30: Travel/Backache 62 • Week 31: Dealing with Discomfort 64 • Week 32: Positions for Labour 66 • Week 33: Emotions in Late Pregnancy 68 • Week 34: Older First-time Mothers 70 • Week 35: Final Preparations 72 • Week 36: Discomforts in Late Pregnancy 74 • Week 37: As Birth Approaches 76 • Week 38: Induction/Pain Relief in Labour 78 • Week 39: Complications During Birth 80 • Week 40: Labour and Birth 82 • Post-Natal Care 86

GLOSSARY OF PREGNANCY TERMS 92
INDEX 94
USEFUL ADDRESSES 96

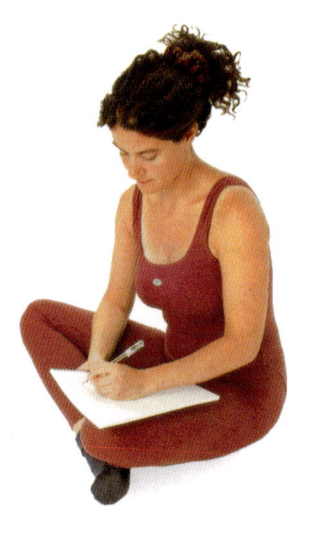

INTRODUCTION

PREGNANCY IS A VERY SPECIAL TIME for both you and your partner. Knowing what is happening to you and your growing baby during the weeks ahead will help you both to enjoy this exciting period in your lives. Starting with pre-conceptual care, this book explains how conception takes place and then looks at pregnancy and your baby's development week by week. Many of the issues raised will be relevant throughout your pregnancy and not just during the week in which they are first mentioned, so do read it all.

It is normal to experience some minor discomforts during pregnancy and you will want to know how to cope with them. More serious problems can occasionally occur, and it is important to recognize the symptoms so that you will know when immediate medical treatment is required. The birth is something you may feel anxious about and it will help you if you understand the choices available in both ante-natal care and childbirth. By being informed you will be able to choose the type of care and birth that is right for you.

As your body adapts to the changes that pregnancy brings, you will begin to prepare yourself physically, emotionally and practically for parenthood. A well-balanced, healthy diet is essential for both your well-being and that of your baby. Exercise has an important part to play too, not just in keeping you fit but also in preparing your body for the birth. Looking good will help you to feel good, so you should take care of your physical appearance throughout your pregnancy. Knowing how to select the right clothes to suit your changing shape and how to use make-up to emphasize your best features will help you to feel confident and make your pregnancy an even more enjoyable experience.

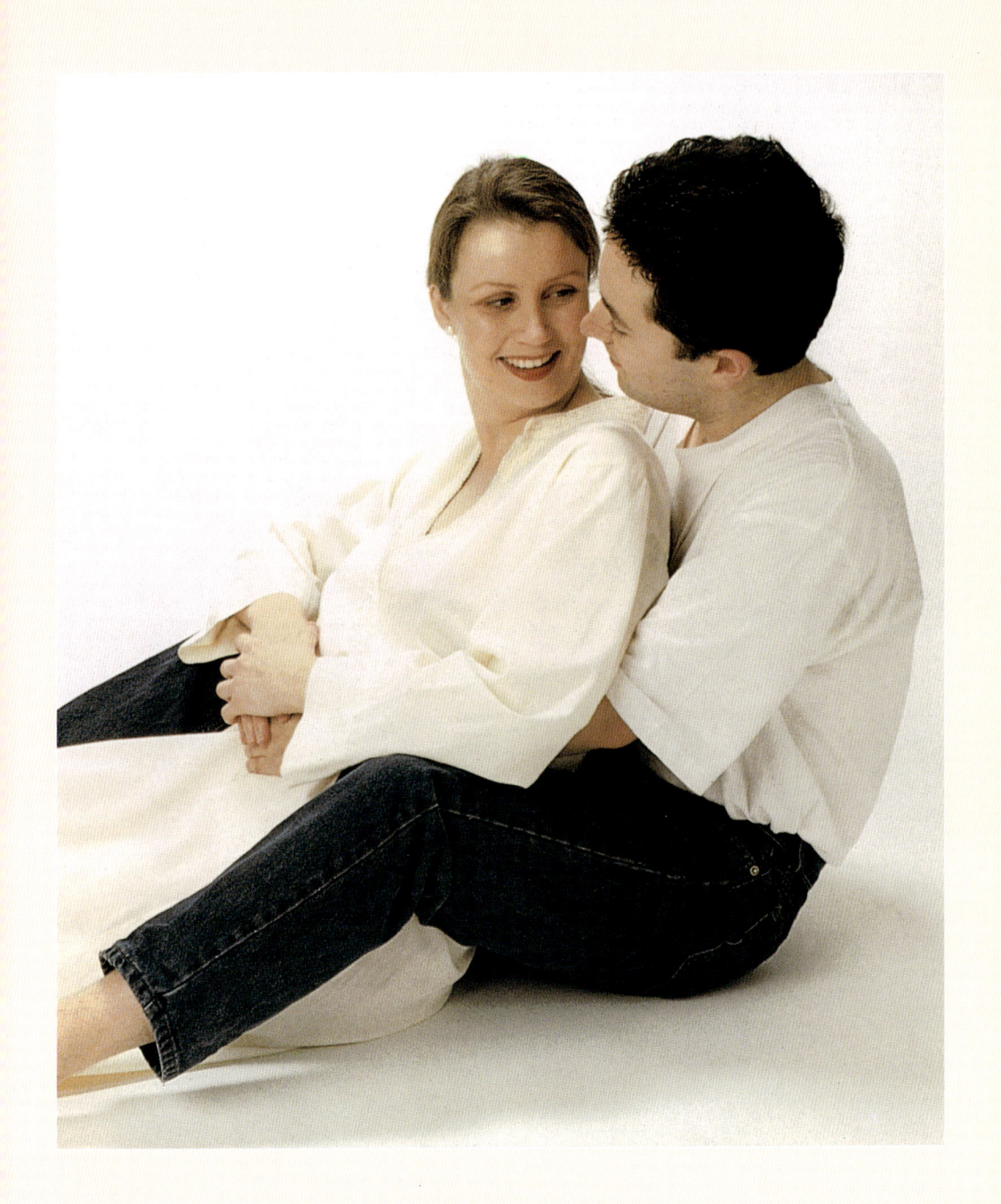

PREPARING FOR PREGNANCY

Once you have decided that you want to have a baby, you and your partner should concentrate on getting yourselves fit and healthy before you try to conceive. Ideally, you should begin preparing for pregnancy at least three months before conception so that you can be sure that your child will get the best possible start in life. If your pregnancy is unplanned, then start taking extra care of yourself as soon as you suspect that you might be pregnant. This may involve some basic changes in your lifestyle.

There is evidence that suggests that smoking by either partner can delay conception, so if you or your partner smoke you should stop now. In addition, smoking during pregnancy will put the baby at risk and can also affect your well-being; giving up before conception will benefit you and your child.

Alcohol can inhibit fertility, so both you and your partner should avoid drinking alcohol while trying to conceive. Once you are pregnant alcohol can restrict fetal development and could even cause malformation. Since there is no safe limit for alcohol during pregnancy it is better to give it up altogether.

Medication
Fertilization and the early development of a baby are controlled by delicately balanced chemical processes in the body. Additional chemicals entering your body as medication can upset this development, so if possible you should avoid taking any medicines before conception and during pregnancy. If you are on long-term medication, you will need to talk to your doctor about alternatives. Medicines that are available over the counter, natural remedies, and vitamin supplements should also be avoided, unless they have been recommended by your doctor.

Oral contraceptives rely on chemically-produced hormones to control fertility. If you are taking the pill, change to a barrier method, such as the condom or diaphragm, for three months before trying to conceive. This allows your body to clear itself of synthetic hormones and to re-establish its own cycle.

Immunizations
An unborn baby exposed to rubella (German measles) during its early development can be born severely handicapped. Don't assume that because you were vaccinated in your teens, or you have had the infection, that you are automatically immune. Ask your doctor to give you a blood

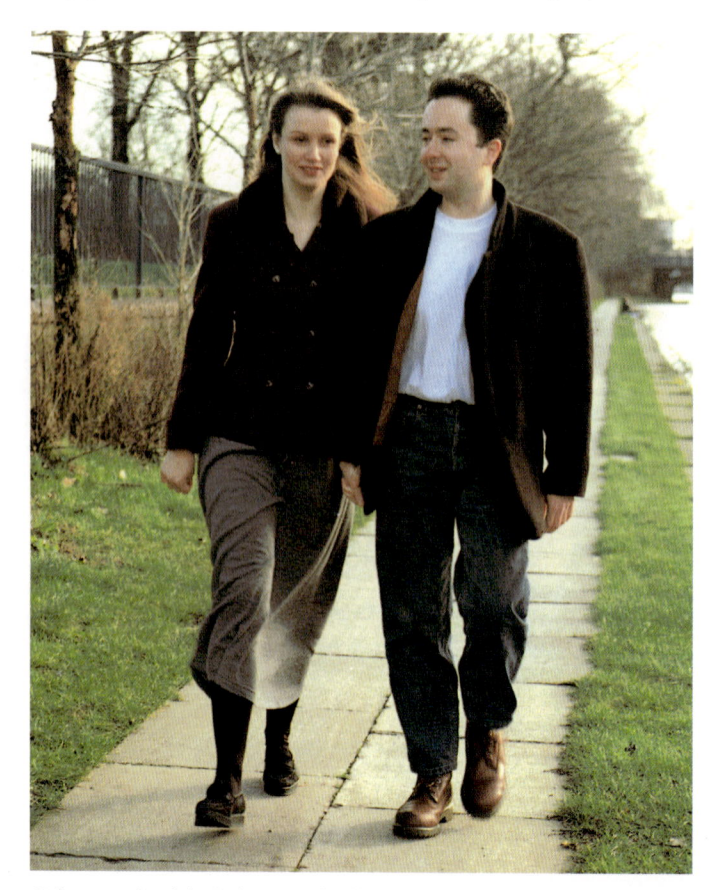

Before trying for a baby, both partners should try to get fit by walking and other exercise.

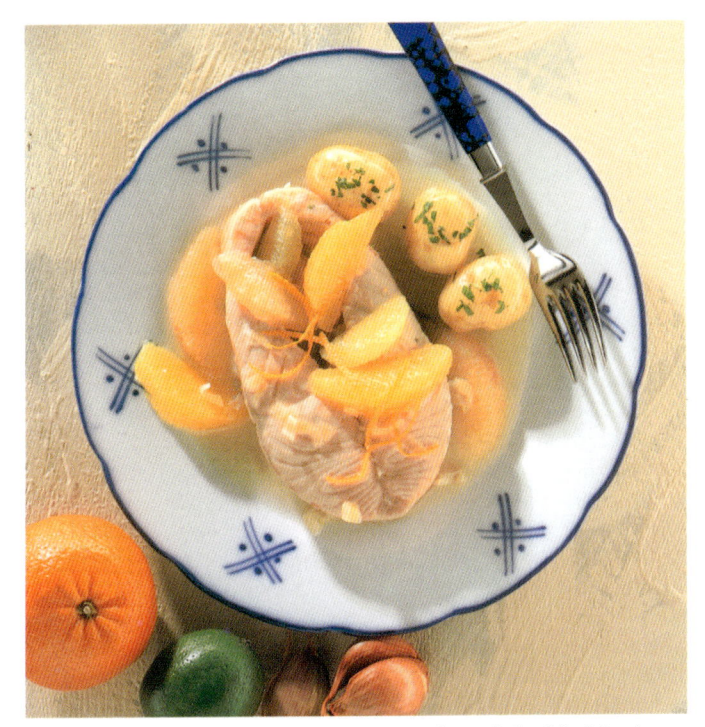

Salmon is ideal as part of a balanced diet, because it is low in fat but full of vitamins.

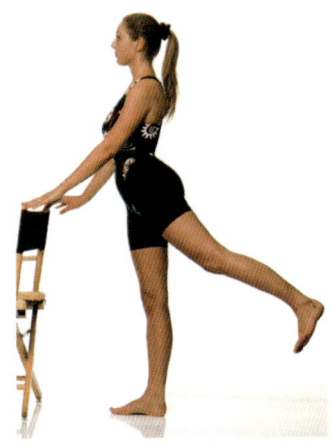

By doing regular stretching exercises at home, or at an organized class, you will strengthen yourself for pregnancy.

test to check. If you are not immune you can be vaccinated, but you should not get pregnant until the vaccine virus has cleared from your blood, which takes about three months. If you have been given vaccines for tropical diseases, you should also wait for three months before getting pregnant.

NUTRITION AND EXERCISE

A well-balanced, healthy diet that contains reasonable daily amounts of carbohydrate, protein, fat, minerals, and vitamins is essential for both your well-being and that of your baby. Everything you eat will also become your unborn child's nourishment, and what you store before pregnancy is important for early fetal development when all the major organs are formed.

One of the B vitamins, folic acid, helps prevent neural tube defects (NTD), such as spina bifida, in unborn babies. It is recommended that all women planning a pregnancy should increase their average daily intake to 0.6 mg by taking a 0.4 mg supplement before attempting conception, and during the first 12 weeks of pregnancy. This is the time when your baby's organs and body systems are forming.

Regular exercise, such as brisk walking or swimming, is important if you are to maintain a healthy lifestyle. Exercise will help you get fit before conception and, as your pregnancy progresses, it will strengthen muscles in your lower back, stomach, and legs, which will help your body cope better with the demands of pregnancy.

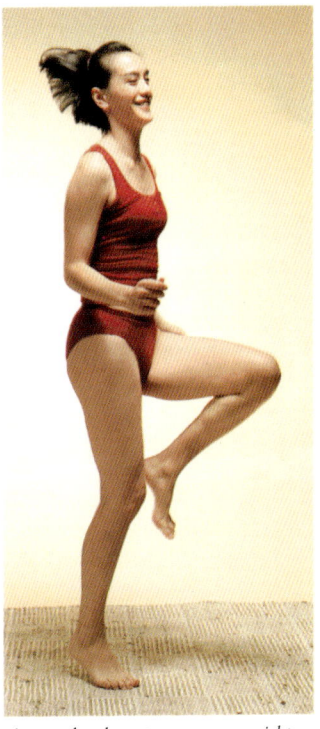

As your legs have to carry more weight during pregnancy, try to do regular daily exercises such as running on the spot to build them up.

WEEKS 1-4: CONCEPTION

THE FIRST TRIMESTER

WEEKS 1–4: CONCEPTION

You and your body
You won't be aware of the changes that are happening inside your body during these early weeks, although it is possible that you may experience very slight bleeding at the time when your next period would have been due. Usually the first indication that you are pregnant will be a missed period.

During the first half of the menstrual cycle two chemical substances called hormones are released from special glands into the bloodstream. One hormone stimulates the process that results in the production of an ovum, or ripe egg. The other hormone stimulates the endometrium, or lining of the uterus (womb), to thicken in readiness to receive a fertilized ovum. About two weeks from the end of your menstrual cycle the work of the first hormone is completed and you ovulate; that is, a ripe ovum is released from one of your ovaries. Conception occurs if your partner's sperm fertilizes this ovum. This usually takes place in the Fallopian tube that connects the ovary to the uterus. The fertilized ovum completes its journey to the uterus, where it implants into the thickened uterine lining. Once this process occurs the cervix increases slightly in width and becomes softer, and a thick mucous plug seals off the uterus to protect it from infection. After two weeks, if there has been no conception, the thickened uterine lining is shed and menstruation takes place.

AFTER FERTILIZATION
The fertilized single-cell egg multiplies into two, then four cells, and it carries on multiplying so that by about day seven, when it reaches the uterus, it has grown into a ball of over 100 cells with a fluid-filled cavity. This ball, called a blastocyst, has two layers: the outer one becomes the placenta, while the inner one forms the embryo, which develops into your baby.

The embryo is made up of three layers of tissue, each of which forms separately. The outer layer develops into the nerves and skin; the middle layer forms the bones, cartilage, muscles, circulatory system, kidneys, and sex organs; and the inner layer becomes the respiratory and digestive systems.

The placenta is the unborn baby's life-support system. It is attached to the lining of the uterus and separates the developing baby's circulation

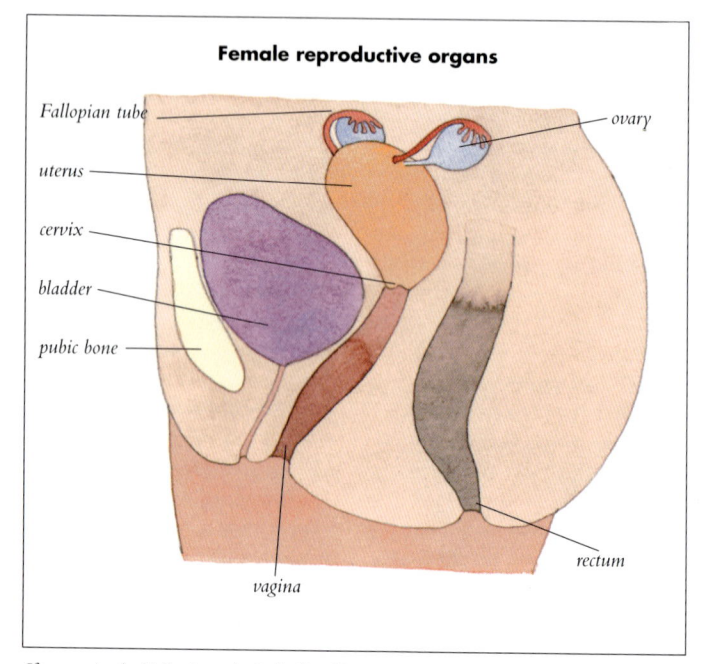

Female reproductive organs

Fallopian tube
uterus
cervix
bladder
pubic bone
ovary
rectum
vagina

If an egg in the Fallopian tube is fertilized by a sperm, it will embed itself into the lining of the uterus. If not, it is shed down through the cervix and out through the vagina.

10

Weeks 1-4: Conception

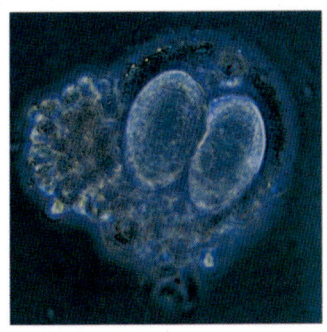

This fertilized egg now has two cells called blastomeres and is the primitive embryo. It will multiply to over 100 cells.

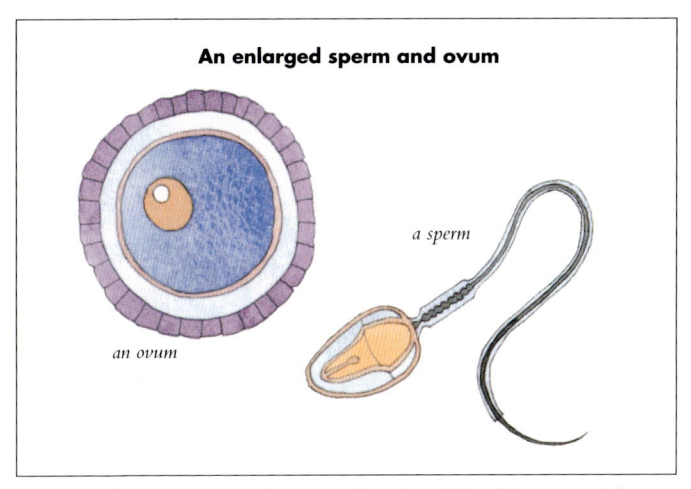

An enlarged sperm and ovum

an ovum

a sperm

A sperm and an ovum are tiny. A man ejaculates about 500 million sperm, while a woman usually produces one ovum half-way through her menstrual cycle.

from its mother's. It allows oxygen and food, as well as protective antibodies, to pass from the mother along the umbilical cord to the baby. The placenta isn't fully formed until the end of the 12th week of pregnancy when it is able to take over the production of the pregnancy hormones, oestrogen and progesterone, from the ovaries.

Within the uterus, the embryo is contained in the amniotic sac. This is filled with fluid in which the developing child will float until birth. The amniotic fluid offers protection from any external pressures.

THE BABY'S SEX

A child's sex is determined by the father's sperm at the time of conception. Sperm carry either an X or Y chromosome while the egg has only an X chromosome. If a Y-chromosome sperm fertilizes the egg, the baby will be a boy. If the sperm carries an X chromosome, the baby will be a girl.

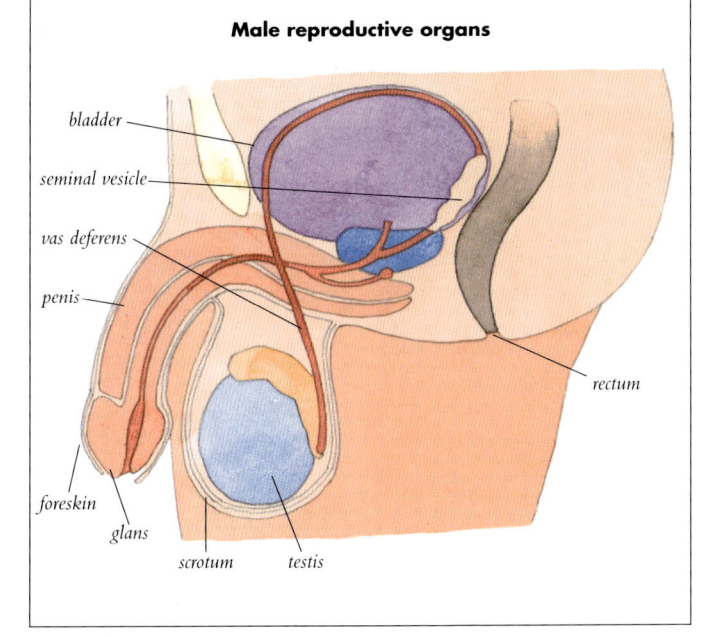

Male reproductive organs

- bladder
- seminal vesicle
- vas deferens
- penis
- foreskin
- glans
- scrotum
- testis
- rectum

Sperm mature in both testes. When a man is sexually aroused, the penis becomes erect and the outlet from the bladder into the ejaculatory duct is closed leaving it free for sperm.

Trimesters

Pregnancy lasts approximately 40 weeks and is calculated from the first day of your last period, although conception will probably not have taken place until around two weeks after this. Pregnancy is divided into three parts known as trimesters. The first covers weeks 1–13, the second trimester weeks 14–26, and the third trimester week 27 until birth.

WEEK 5: CONFIRMING PREGNANCY

Pregnancy can be confirmed by means of a simple test that measures the levels of the pregnancy hormone, human chorionic gonadotrophin (HCG), that are present in your urine. The test can be carried out as soon as you reach the day that your next period should have started. Your doctor or Family Planning Clinic will do the test free, or you may prefer to carry out a home test yourself using one of the kits available from the pharmacist. Ensure that you choose a kit that will give an accurate result this early. Although many modern home-testing kits state that you can test your urine at any time, you may wish to use an early morning sample because this urine will contain the highest concentration of HCG.

If the result is positive, you must make an appointment to see your doctor so that he or she can make arrangements for your ante-natal care and the birth.

EARLY SYMPTOMS

Some women experience all the early symptoms of pregnancy, while others sail through the first weeks without any feelings of discomfort.
- Your body is having to work hard to adapt to the demands of pregnancy, so you may feel overwhelmingly tired. Try to get as much rest as possible. You will find that sitting with your feet up for even half an hour will help.
- Your breasts may tingle or feel tender, rather as they do before a period; your nipples will appear darker and more prominent and the veins will be more noticeable. You should wear a good support bra from now until after your baby is born.
- You may experience a strange metallic taste in the mouth, which

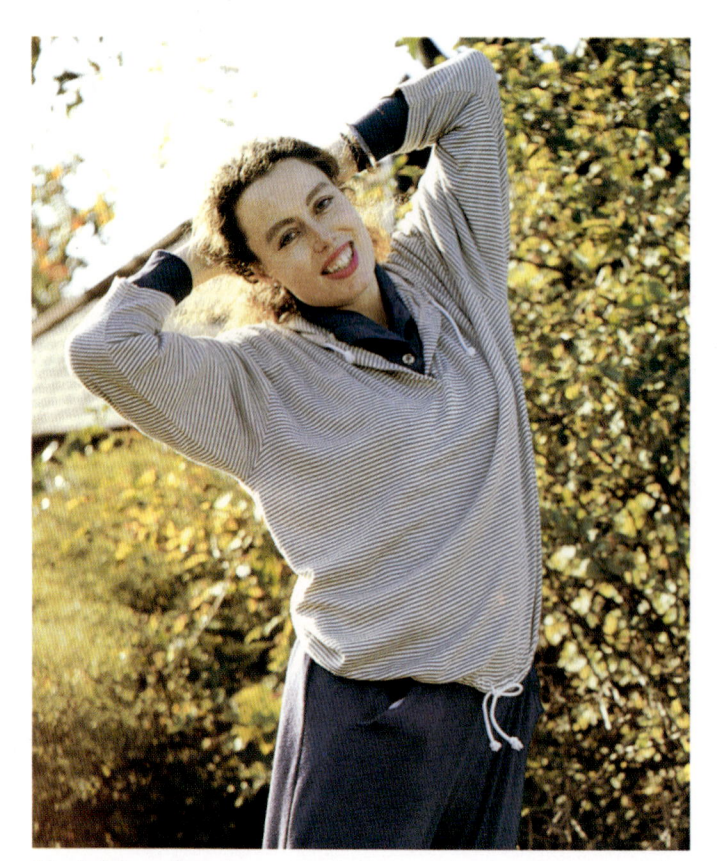

If you're lucky, you'll experience no nausea in pregnancy and continue exercising as normal.

Your growing baby
Although the embryo is only just visible to the naked eye, the spinal column and brain have already begun to grow and a blood vessel has developed which will become the heart. The embryo is 4 mm/⅛ in long.

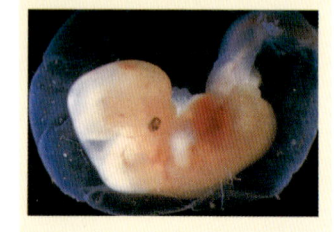

You and your body
This is the first week that you will be able to confirm that you are pregnant.

WEEK 5: CONFIRMING PREGNANCY

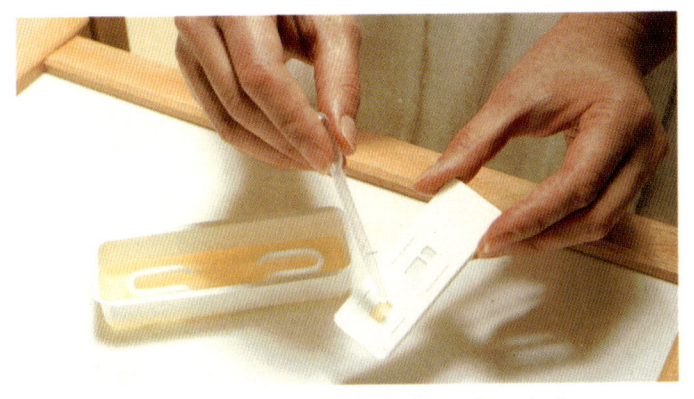

To confirm a pregnancy, you can do a test with a kit from a pharmacist, but ensure you choose one that is suitable to use for a test at five weeks.

can be accompanied by going off certain foods and tea and coffee.
• A feeling of nausea, or even actual physical sickness in the morning or at any time during the day, is quite usual. It is often worse when your stomach is empty, so have a plain biscuit and a cup of tea before you get up in the morning. During the day try eating six high-carbohydrate meals, such as pasta, potato, and bread. Avoid rich or fatty foods.
• Finally, as the enlarging uterus presses on your bladder you may need to urinate more frequently.

DATING THE BIRTH

Once your pregnancy is confirmed, you will want to know your baby's likely date of birth. You can calculate an estimated date of delivery (EDD) by counting 40 weeks from the first day of your last period. But you should remember that since you don't know the exact date of ovulation this EDD is approximate. At about 10 weeks you may be offered an ultrasound scan to confirm the EDD.

Estimated date of delivery

JANUARY	1	2	3	4	5	6	7	8	9	10	11	12	13	14	15	16	17	18	19	20	21	22	23	24	25	26	27	28	29	30	31	JANUARY
OCTOBER	8	9	10	11	12	13	14	15	16	17	18	19	20	21	22	23	24	25	26	27	28	29	30	31	1	2	3	4	5	6	7	NOVEMBER
FEBRUARY	1	2	3	4	5	6	7	8	9	10	11	12	13	14	15	16	17	18	19	20	21	22	23	24	25	26	27	28				FEBRUARY
NOVEMBER	8	9	10	11	12	13	14	15	16	17	18	19	20	21	22	23	24	25	26	27	28	29	30	1	2	3	4	5				DECEMBER
MARCH	1	2	3	4	5	6	7	8	9	10	11	12	13	14	15	16	17	18	19	20	21	22	23	24	25	26	27	28	29	30	31	MARCH
DECEMBER	6	7	8	9	10	11	12	13	14	15	16	17	18	19	20	21	22	23	24	25	26	27	28	29	30	31	1	2	3	4	5	JANUARY
APRIL	1	2	3	4	5	6	7	8	9	10	11	12	13	14	15	16	17	18	19	20	21	22	23	24	25	26	27	28	29	30		APRIL
JANUARY	6	7	8	9	10	11	12	13	14	15	16	17	18	19	20	21	22	23	24	25	26	27	28	29	30	31	1	2	3	4		FEBRUARY
MAY	1	2	3	4	5	6	7	8	9	10	11	12	13	14	15	16	17	18	19	20	21	22	23	24	25	26	27	28	29	30	31	MAY
FEBRUARY	5	6	7	8	9	10	11	12	13	14	15	16	17	18	19	20	21	22	23	24	25	26	27	28	1	2	3	4	5	6	7	MARCH
JUNE	1	2	3	4	5	6	7	8	9	10	11	12	13	14	15	16	17	18	19	20	21	22	23	24	25	26	27	28	29	30		JUNE
MARCH	8	9	10	11	12	13	14	15	16	17	18	19	20	21	22	23	24	25	26	27	28	29	30	31	1	2	3	4	5	6		APRIL
JULY	1	2	3	4	5	6	7	8	9	10	11	12	13	14	15	16	17	18	19	20	21	22	23	24	25	26	27	28	29	30	31	JULY
APRIL	7	8	9	10	11	12	13	14	15	16	17	18	19	20	21	22	23	24	25	26	27	28	29	30	1	2	3	4	5	6	7	MAY
AUGUST	1	2	3	4	5	6	7	8	9	10	11	12	13	14	15	16	17	18	19	20	21	22	23	24	25	26	27	28	29	30	31	AUGUST
MAY	8	9	10	11	12	13	14	15	16	17	18	19	20	21	22	23	24	25	26	27	28	29	30	31	1	2	3	4	5	6	7	JUNE
SEPTEMBER	1	2	3	4	5	6	7	8	9	10	11	12	13	14	15	16	17	18	19	20	21	22	23	24	25	26	27	28	29	30		SEPTEMBER
JUNE	8	9	10	11	12	13	14	15	16	17	18	19	20	21	22	23	24	25	26	27	28	29	30	1	2	3	4	5	6	7		JULY
OCTOBER	1	2	3	4	5	6	7	8	9	10	11	12	13	14	15	16	17	18	19	20	21	22	23	24	25	26	27	28	29	30	31	OCTOBER
JULY	8	9	10	11	12	13	14	15	16	17	18	19	20	21	22	23	24	25	26	27	28	29	30	31	1	2	3	4	5	6	7	AUGUST
NOVEMBER	1	2	3	4	5	6	7	8	9	10	11	12	13	14	15	16	17	18	19	20	21	22	23	24	25	26	27	28	29	30		NOVEMBER
AUGUST	8	9	10	11	12	13	14	15	16	17	18	19	20	21	22	23	24	25	26	27	28	29	30	31	1	2	3	4	5	6		SEPTEMBER
DECEMBER	1	2	3	4	5	6	7	8	9	10	11	12	13	14	15	16	17	18	19	20	21	22	23	24	25	26	27	28	29	30	31	DECEMBER
SEPTEMBER	7	8	9	10	11	12	13	14	15	16	17	18	19	20	21	22	23	24	25	26	27	28	29	30	1	2	3	4	5	6	7	OCTOBER

Find the first day of your last period on the white bands; the date on the tint band below is your EDD.

WEEK 6: ANTE-NATAL CHOICES

Who looks after you, and where your ante-natal care takes place, will depend a lot on the type of birth you want to have. If you decide on a home birth, the care will be carried out at home by a midwife and at your doctor's surgery. If you want a hospital birth your care will probably be shared between a midwife, your doctor and the hospital.

If you are not registered with a doctor, or you want a home birth but your particular doctor doesn't want to assist in the delivery, or you would rather be seen by a woman doctor and your doctor is a man, you can go to see a different doctor just for your maternity care.

The actual care you get will be similar wherever you receive it, because all ante-natal care is designed to ensure that you and your unborn baby remain healthy during pregnancy.

These days, the best pattern of ante-natal care for a healthy woman is considered to be no more than nine ante-natal appointments. If you have any concerns between these appointments, you can telephone your midwife or doctor for advice.

HOME BIRTH
A home birth means you give birth in the familiar surroundings of your own home under the supervision of a midwife. If you want to deliver your baby in this way, you will need to talk to your doctor to see whether there are any medical reasons why this isn't advisable. It is also a good idea to contact the director of maternity services (or local supervisor of midwives) at your hospital in order to arrange for a midwife to

You and your body
If you are suffering from morning sickness, you may find that the smell of certain things, such as tobacco smoke or frying food, brings on the sickness or makes it worse. The texture of your skin may become dry and flaky, or you may get spots. Now is the time to start thinking about your ante-natal care, and the type of birth you want.

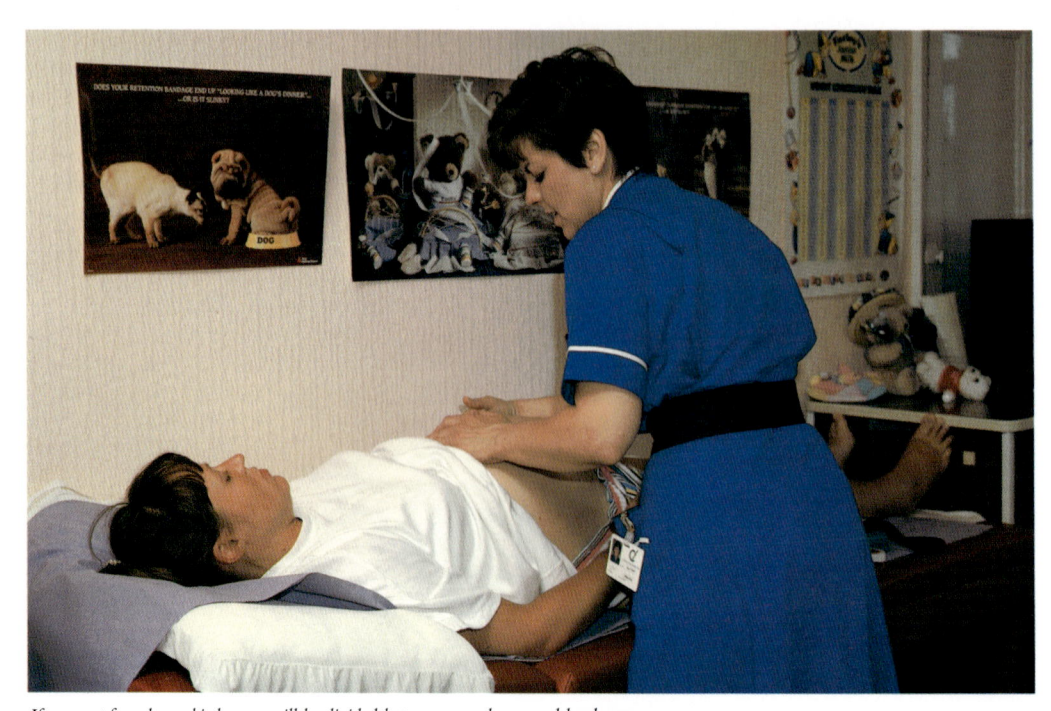

If you opt for a home birth, care will be divided between your home and local surgery.

come and visit you and discuss a home delivery in detail.

HOSPITAL BIRTH
Some women prefer a hospital birth because they feel safer knowing that there will be experts on hand to help if there are any complications. Also, if the baby needs special care this will be available almost immediately. Although hospitals are no longer the dictatorial places they used to be, and most try to cater for parents' wishes, not all of them are able to offer every type of birth. You will need to find out what facilities your local hospital offers. Before making your final decision talk to other mothers who have had their babies there recently. If you have any worries, discuss these with your doctor.

There are a number of hospital birth schemes that involve your doctor and midwife to varying degrees:
Midwife unit This is usually based at the hospital and is run entirely by midwives who undertake ante-natal care, delivery and post-natal care. You can choose to have your baby at home or in the unit. These units are not widely available throughout the country, so this may not be an option that is open to you.
Domino scheme The Domino scheme (Domiciliary Midwife In and Out) means that your doctor and community midwife look after you throughout your pregnancy. Once you are in labour the midwife comes to your home and stays with you until you are ready to go into hospital. She then accompanies you to the hospital you are booked into, where she delivers the baby. You can usually return home around six hours after the birth. The midwife then continues to look after you at your home. Many women like the continuity this scheme gives them, but unfortunately it is not available in all areas at the present time.
Shared care Your ante-natal care will be shared between your doctor and the hospital where your baby is going to be born. The birth will take place in the maternity unit of this hospital and your doctor and midwife will look after you jointly on your return home with your young baby.

PRIVATE CARE
If you can afford it, you may like to consider having a home birth with a private, or independent, midwife taking care of you. She will provide all your ante-natal and post-natal care and will also deliver your baby.

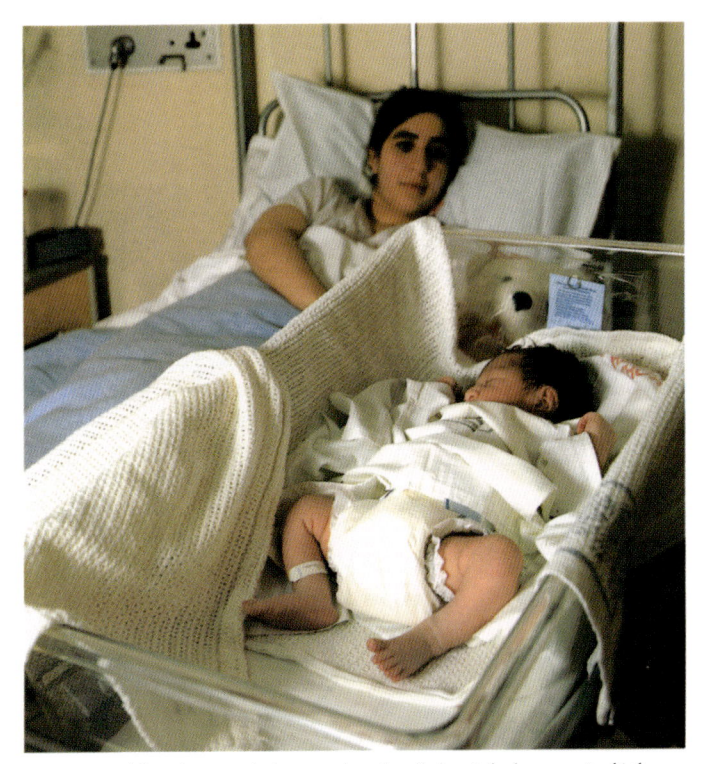

You can spend from between six hours to three days in hospital when you give birth, depending on your delivery. After the birth you may keep your baby beside you.

Alternatively, you can decide to have your baby in a private hospital or maternity home.

Your growing baby
The heart has now formed in the chest cavity and is beginning to beat. By the end of this week the stalk connecting the embryo to the placenta will have begun to grow into the umbilical cord and blood vessels will have started to form. The embryo is now about the size of your little fingernail and its movements can be picked up by ultrasound scan. The head has the beginning of the eyes, ears, and mouth and there are tiny buds which will become arms and legs.

WEEK 7: POSSIBLE PROBLEMS

Although the majority of pregnancies go without a hitch, sometimes serious problems do occur and special care is needed. Complications can usually be resolved with monitoring, but occasionally the pregnancy comes to an end. Although the following conditions are not likely to affect you, you should be aware of their symptoms:

Pre-eclampsia This is a high blood pressure condition that can occur during pregnancy. If pre-eclampsia is left untreated it causes the blood vessels of the placenta to spasm, which reduces the oxygen flow to the fetus and puts it at risk; the fetal growth rate may also be affected. Symptoms include oedema, which is fluid retention causing swelling of the hands, feet, and ankles, protein in the urine and a sudden increase in weight. You will be tested for signs of pre-eclampsia at each ante-natal check. In the early stages pre-eclampsia is treated with complete bed-rest under medical supervision. Later in the pregnancy, if the condition is severe, it may become necessary to induce the birth as early as it is safe to do so. The mother's blood pressure will soon return to normal. If the condition is left completely untreated it can develop into eclampsia, which can be fatal for both mother and child. Today, this condition is extremely rare.

Bleeding in early pregnancy
Bleeding or spotting from the vagina is known as a threatened miscarriage. It is possible to bleed quite heavily and not miscarry or do any harm to the baby. All bleeding in pregnancy must be taken seriously, however, and you should report it to your doctor immediately. Your doctor is likely to carry out an internal pelvic examination and arrange for you to have an ultrasound scan to see whether the baby is developing normally. Providing everything is all right you will probably be told to rest until the bleeding stops.

Ectopic pregnancy This occurs when the fertilized egg implants itself in one of the Fallopian tubes rather than in the uterus. If it is undetected, the growing baby eventually ruptures the tube.

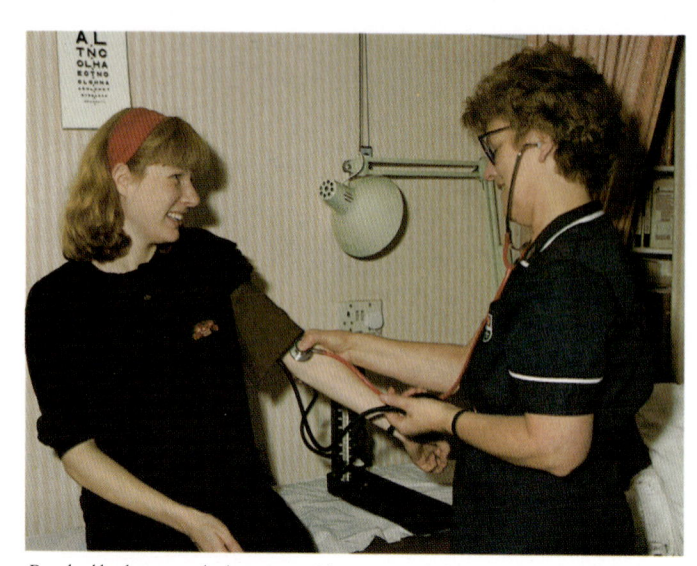

Regular blood pressure checks are essential at ante-natal clinics to detect pre-eclampsia.

You and your body

You may feel dizzy or even faint if you stand for too long or you are in a crowd. Overwhelming tiredness can also be a problem now, so make sure you get plenty of rest. If you don't feel like making love at the moment don't worry; this is quite normal and you may find that your sex life is better then ever in the second trimester.

Your growing baby

The unborn baby is now known as a fetus and is about 1.3 cm/½ in long. The nostrils, lips, tongue, and teeth are beginning to form and the arms and legs are growing. Lungs are beginning to develop and the intestines, spine, and brain are almost fully developed.

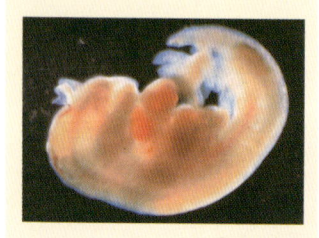

Week 7: Possible Problems

Immediate surgery is required to terminate the pregnancy, and this often means losing the Fallopian tube as well. In extreme cases the ovary may also have to be removed. If the other ovary and Fallopian tube are healthy, there is no reason why another successful pregnancy should not take place. If the ectopic pregnancy is discovered early enough, a drug can be given that causes the embryo to be reabsorbed by the body; this prevents the Fallopian tube from bursting. Symptoms of an ectopic pregnancy include pain in the side of the abdomen, vaginal bleeding, and fainting.

Miscarriage The most common time for miscarriage is during the first three months of pregnancy, although losing a baby at any time before the 24th week is described as a miscarriage. Some miscarriages occur for no known reason. Known causes of miscarriage include hormonal problems, disease or infection, abnormalities of the uterus, or an incompetent cervix. If this last condition is known to exist, it can be dealt with by a simple surgical suture that will be removed shortly before the EDD.

Although it is unlikely that sexual intercourse will cause miscarriage, women who have experienced bleeding early in their pregnancy or who are known to have a tendency to miscarry are usually advised by doctors not to have intercourse for the first 12 weeks, until their pregnancy is well established.

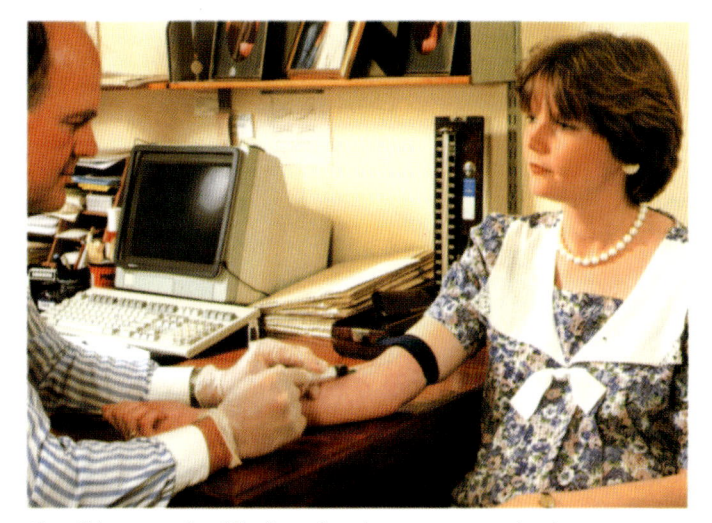

You will have a number of blood tests throughout your pregnancy but these are no cause for alarm. The tests are simply a means for your doctor to make sure that you are progressing normally and not experiencing any problems.

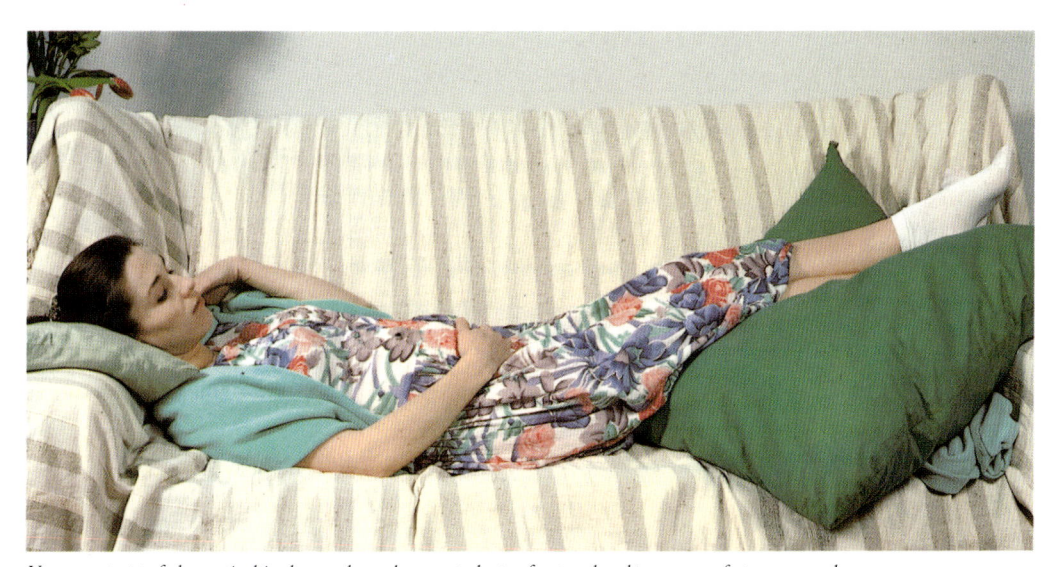

You may start to feel very tired in these early weeks, so get plenty of rest and make sure your feet are propped up.

WEEK 8: BOOKING-IN/ROUTINE TESTS

Your first ante-natal check-up will take place between eight and 12 weeks, either at your doctor's surgery or at the hospital where you plan to give birth. This first visit is usually referred to as the booking-in clinic. You will be asked a lot of personal questions about your health, family medical history, and possibly even about your and your partner's jobs and living accommodation. All this information is required to build up a picture of you and your pregnancy so that any potential risks can be spotted and help can be offered where needed.

If you have any questions or worries, this is a good time to discuss them. It's easy to forget to ask something important when there is so much to take in at one time, so it may help to write down things that you want to know about before you attend the clinic.

ROUTINE TESTS

Certain tests are carried out during pregnancy to ensure that both you and the fetus are progressing well. Some of these will be repeated at each ante-natal visit; others are only carried out at the booking-in clinic.

Blood pressure This will be taken at each visit. Increased blood pressure could develop into pre-eclampsia, which could endanger both you and the fetus.

Urine You will be asked to bring a sample of urine with you to each ante-natal visit. This will be tested for any infections that may require some treatment, as well as for sugar, protein, or the chemical substances known as ketones. Sugar in the urine could be a sign of diabetes; protein may indicate the onset of pre-eclampsia; and ketones may indicate that your kidneys are being adversely affected by your pregnancy.

You and your body

The changes to your body are becoming more noticeable as your breasts and nipples enlarge and become sensitive. Your vagina changes from light to dark pink, and you may notice an increased vaginal discharge.

It is time for regular monitoring of your pregnancy.

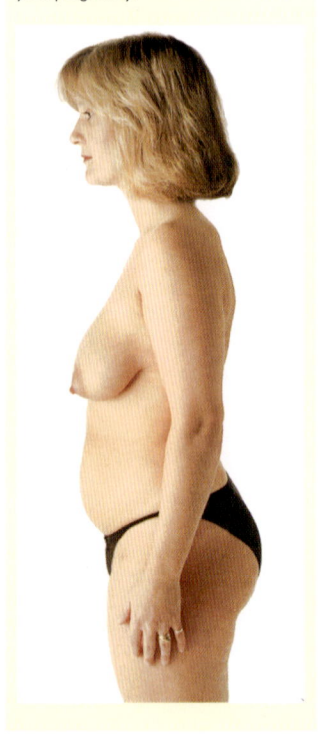

Weight gain during pregnancy

Baby 39%
Blood 22%
Amniotic fluid 11%
Uterus 11%
Placenta 9%
Breasts 8%

Your weight increases by about ½–1 kg/1–2 lb weekly during months four to eight, with very little in the last month. As your breasts get larger, the uterus, placenta and baby develop, and the amniotic fluid increases, until they reach the percentages shown here.

The amount of weight that you will gain during pregnancy varies, depending on your height and size, but can be as much as 19 kg/40 lb.

Weight Your weight may be monitored regularly to see how the baby is growing, although not all doctors do this. You can expect to gain anything from 6 kg to 19 kg/20 lb to 40 lb during your pregnancy, with most of this extra weight going on after the 20th week. A sudden increase in weight could be an indication of pre-eclampsia.

Height You will be measured at your first appointment because

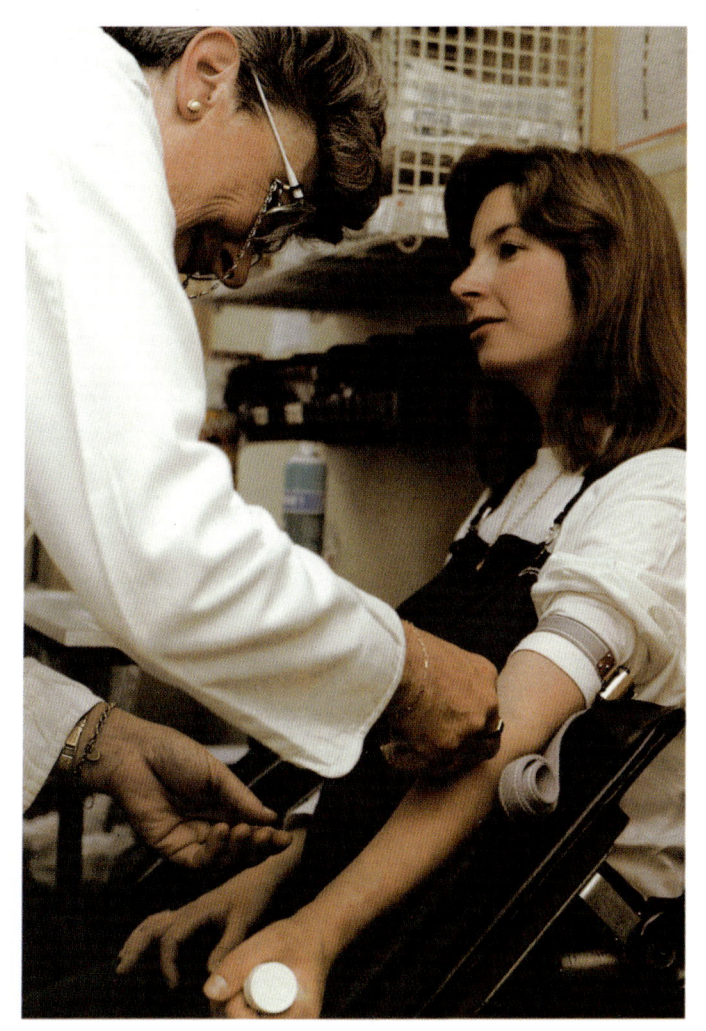

At your first ante-natal check-up, a blood sample will be taken to find out your blood group and type, and to make sure you're not anaemic or carrying a virus such as hepatitis B. You will have blood tests regularly through your pregnancy.

your height gives a rough guide to the size of your pelvis. If your pelvis is too small to accommodate your baby's head at the birth, then a Caesarean delivery may be indicated. It is worth noting, however, that most babies are in proportion to the mothers who carry them.

Blood tests At your first appointment you will be asked to give a blood sample to confirm your blood group and to find out if you are rhesus negative or positive.

Your blood will also be checked to see if you are anaemic and if you are immune to rubella (German measles). Other tests are also carried out to detect any serious conditions that could affect your baby, such as syphilis and hepatitis B. If you are of Afro-Caribbean descent, they will test your blood for sickle-cell disease; if you are of a Mediterranean ethnic group they will test for thalassaemia.

Sometimes your blood will also be tested anonymously to see if the HIV or AIDS virus is present.

Internal examination You may have an internal examination at your booking-in clinic. This is to check for any abnormalities of the vagina, cervix, or uterus. If you haven't had a cervical smear test during the last three to five years you may well be given one.

Wrists and ankles These will be checked at each visit for swelling, or oedema, caused by fluid retention, since these signs could possibly indicate pre-eclampsia.

Palpation The doctor or midwife will palpate, that is press, your abdomen to feel the top of the uterus (fundus). He or she will then feel down towards the pelvis to check the size of the fetus and the way it is lying.

Your growing baby

The fetus is now about 2.5 cm/ 1 in long, which is 10,000 times bigger than at conception. All the major organs are present, although still developing. The ears and eyes have formed and the skin covering the eyes will eventually split to form the eyelids. The middle ear, which controls balance as well as hearing, is also developing. The heart is now pumping with a regular beat, and blood vessels can be seen. As the arms and legs grow longer, the fetus begins to move around and starts to kick, although it is still too small at this stage for you to be able to feel it.

WEEK 9: SPECIAL TESTS

Your blood will have been tested at your booking-in appointment to determine your blood group and to establish its rhesus (Rh) status. The rhesus status of your blood depends on whether or not it possesses the rhesus factor. If the factor is present, your blood is Rh-positive, if it is absent, your blood is Rh-negative. Most people's blood is Rh-positive.

If both you and the baby's father are Rh-negative, there is not a problem. Complications only occur when the father's blood is Rh-positive and yours is Rh-negative. The unborn baby may acquire the rhesus factor from its father, which can result in its blood being incompatible with yours. This can lead to a serious or even fatal illness for the baby before, or after the birth. Fortunately, this rarely affects a first pregnancy and it can be prevented in subsequent pregnancies by injections of anti-D gamma globulin, an antibody that may be given during pregnancy and again within 72 hours of a baby being delivered.

SPECIAL TESTS
There are a number of ante-natal tests that are used in special circumstances and usually only when there is some fear of genetic abnormality. They include:

Amniocentesis If you have a family history of genetic abnormalities such as Down's syndrome, cystic fibrosis, or spina bifida, or your blood shows a high or exceptionally low AFP (alpha-fetoprotein) level, you will be offered an amniocentesis usually at around 16–18 weeks. This test is also offered to all women over 35 years of age because they have a higher risk of having a Down's syndrome baby. Guided by ultrasound scan, a long hollow needle is inserted through the wall of the abdomen and the uterus to draw out a sample of amniotic fluid. This is then tested for abnormalities. You will get the results in about four weeks. The test carries a small risk of miscarriage.

Triple/double test The triple test is carried out at 16 weeks to measure the levels of three substances produced by the mother and the placenta. The levels change during pregnancy and a higher level could indicate that the baby may have Down's syndrome or spina bifida. The test cannot confirm that the baby is affected but it does indicate whether further tests, such as amniocentesis, are required. Not all areas use the triple test; some offer the double test, where two substances are measured; other hospitals don't offer the test at all, but you can have it done privately.

Chorionic villus sampling (CVS) CVS is done at around 11 weeks to test for Down's syndrome or other genetic or chromosomal abnormali-

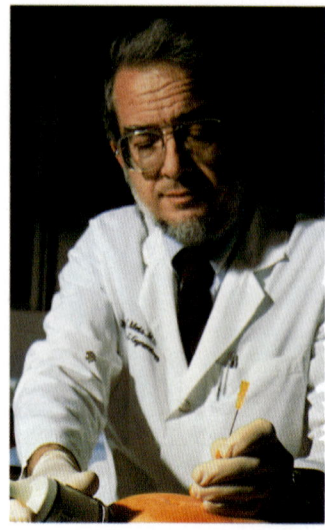

In an amniocentesis test the fetus's position is checked by ultrasound, before amniotic fluid is taken by a needle from the uterus.

Your growing baby
The face is now developing and the mouth and nose are clearly visible. The limbs continue to grow rapidly and the fetus now measures about 3 cm/1¼ in.

You and your body
You will start putting on weight now so it is a good idea to keep a record of any weight gain yourself if your ante-natal care doesn't include regular weight checks. Your gums are becoming softer and thicker because of hormone changes so you will need to pay special attention to oral hygiene.

You should now familiarize yourself with some of the other ante-natal procedures and tests.

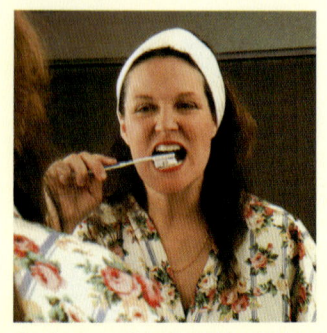

Brush your teeth and gums regularly.

ties. A fine tube is passed into the uterus to remove some of the cells from the tissue that surrounds the baby. The cells are then tested, and the results are usually known within one to two weeks. The advantage of CVS is that if the baby is found to have a problem and you want a termination it can be done early in pregnancy. However, there is a slightly higher risk of miscarriage with CVS than with amniocentesis.

Cordocentesis This test is normally done to confirm diagnosis of chromosomal abnormalities and other handicaps, plus diseases such as rubella and toxoplasmosis. A hollow needle is inserted through the abdomen into the umbilical vein, close to the placenta, and a sample of the baby's blood is withdrawn. It is only performed after 18 weeks when the blood vessels are large enough. Results are usually known within about 48 hours.

GENETIC COUNSELLING

If you are worried about the possibility of your children inheriting a disease or handicap, you can talk to the genetic counsellor who is specially trained to help people with a family history of genetic disorders. Counselling is usually based on details of any genetic diseases that run in the family. A chromosome analysis from a blood sample may also be used. The counsellor will be able to explain the likelihood of future children being affected by the genetic disorder and also about any tests that can be carried out. It is a good idea to have this discussion before attempting to get pregnant so that you know what is involved. Otherwise, tell your doctor that you want to see a genetic counsellor when your pregnancy is confirmed.

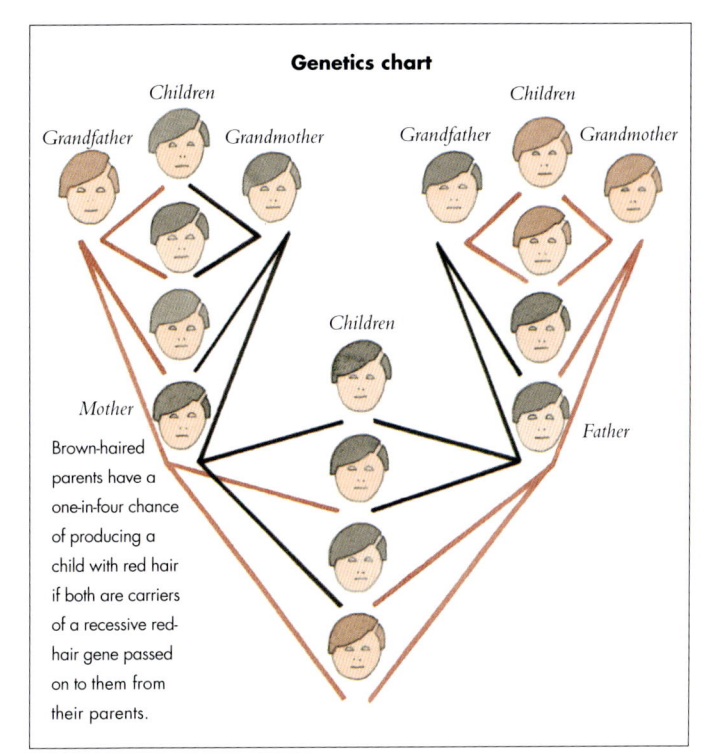

Genetics chart

Brown-haired parents have a one-in-four chance of producing a child with red hair if both are carriers of a recessive red-hair gene passed on to them from their parents.

This genetics chart shows how red hair that is inherited through a recessive gene can miss a generation, but has a high chance of re-appearing in the third generation. This can also apply to some inherited diseases.

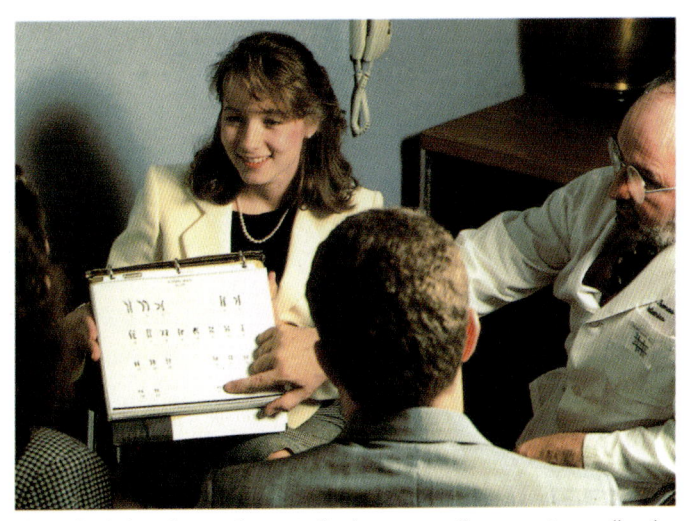

If your family has a history of a genetic disorder, you can talk to a genetic counsellor who will discuss with you and your partner the likelihood of your baby having a problem.

WEEK 10: HORMONES/ MATERNITY RECORD

Hormones play an important part during pregnancy and labour. The prime source of the hormones related to pregnancy are the ovaries during the early stages, and then the placenta once it is established at around 12 weeks. These hormones dictate how fast the fetus grows and are responsible for the changes in your breasts and body. They also ensure that your labour occurs at the right time.

High levels of the hormone called human chorionic gonadotrophin (HCG) circulate in your body during the first 12 weeks of pregnancy. They are responsible for any emotional changes, feeling tired, nausea, and vomiting.

HORMONES AND YOUR EMOTIONS
Pregnancy can produce a number of conflicting emotions, ranging from feelings of pure joy to bouts of black depression. It is quite natural to feel like this as you adjust to your changing role and come to terms with the fact that your life will never be quite the same again. You may find that you start worrying about whether you are ready for motherhood, or the effect that a new baby may have on your established relationship with your partner.

You may also find that mood swings, often brought on by the hormonal changes going on in your body, cause petty arguments between you. So it is most important

You and your body

There is an increase in the amount of blood that is circulating in your body, which may cause you to feel warmer than usual. Your uterus is now the size of a large orange and your changing shape may mean that you are more comfortable in loose-fitting clothes that do not restrict you.

Other changes are also taking place in your body. Although these are not always physically obvious, they are in fact the result of shifts in your body's chemistry.

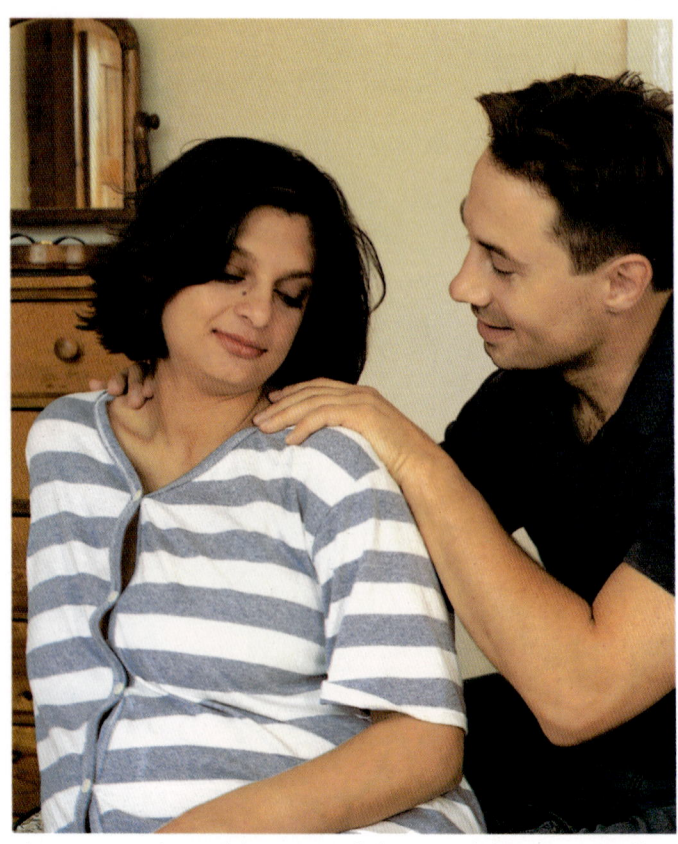

Your growing baby

The external ears are now visible on the head, which is growing fast to make room for the brain. The fetal body is elongating and its fingers and toes are clearly defined but are still joined with webs of skin. At this stage of your pregnancy the fetus is now about 4.5 cm/1¾ in long and weighs around 5 g/¼ oz.

As you experience hormonal changes in your body you may find you become irritable and anxious. Discuss any of your worries with your partner who can talk things through with you and reassure you.

WEEK 10: HORMONES/MATERNITY RECORD

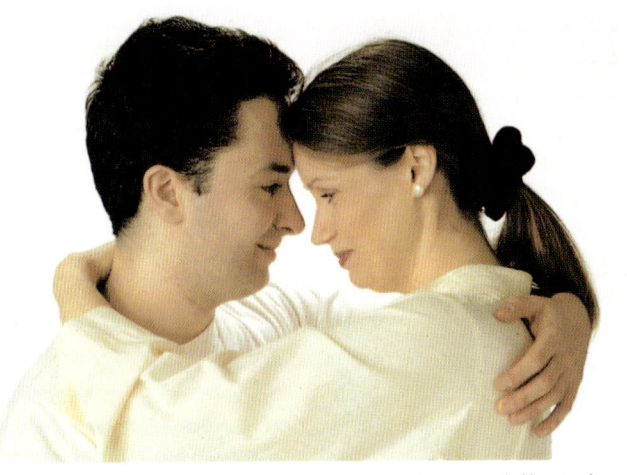

As your emotions are probably mixed up at the moment, don't brood over rows with your partner, but apologize and make up.

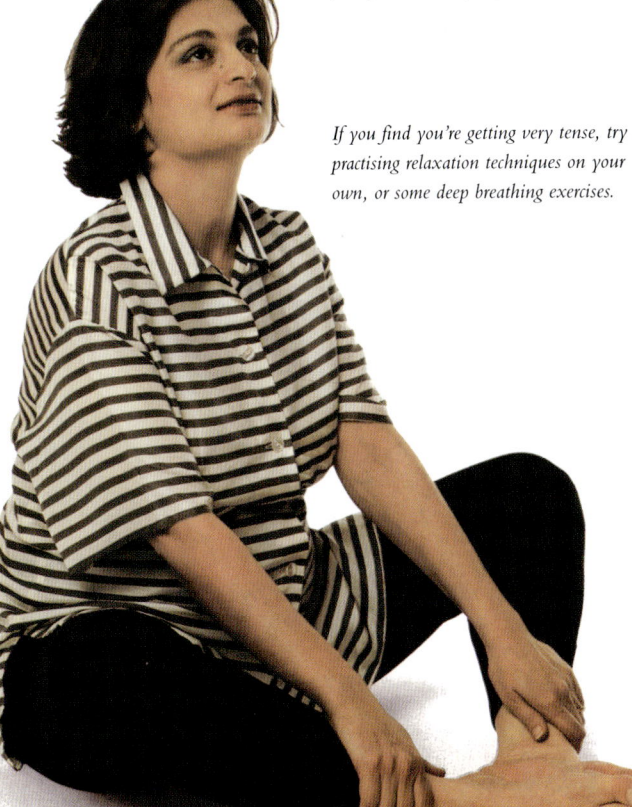

If you find you're getting very tense, try practising relaxation techniques on your own, or some deep breathing exercises.

Terms and abbreviations

The following terms and abbreviations may appear on your maternity record.

AFP: Alpha-fetoprotein.
BP: Blood pressure.
Cephalic: Fetal head is nearest the cervix.
Cx: Cervix.
EDD: Estimated date of delivery.
FHH: Fetal heart heard.
FMF: Fetal movement felt.
Height Fundus: The distance from the pelvis to the top of the uterus is known as the fundus.
LMP: Last menstrual period. This is the date of the first day of your last period before pregnancy.
NAD: No abnormality detected.
Oedema: Swelling of hands and feet because of fluid retention.
Relation of PP to Brim: The position of the fetus's presenting part (PP), that is the part ready to be born first, in relation to the brim of the pelvis.
Transverse: Transverse lie. The fetus is lying across the uterus.
Urine Alb Sugar: Indicates the results of urine tests for protein and sugar.

to make time to talk to each other so that you can both voice your feelings and share any worries or anxieties.

MATERNITY RECORD

You will be given your maternity record card at your booking-in clinic. It is used to record the results of all the tests and examinations that are carried out during your pregnancy. You should keep it with you at all times, so that if you ever need medical attention when you are away from home all the information about your pregnancy is readily available to the medical staff.

WEEK 11: COMMON DISCOMFORTS

As your body prepares itself for birth, you may experience some physical effects. These are perfectly normal, can usually be dealt with easily, and should not leave any long-lasting effects, but knowing the reason for a complaint can often help in dealing with it.

Backache This can occur at any time, but usually happens when you try to compensate for your baby's weight by leaning backwards which puts a strain on the lower back's muscles and joints. Try to avoid lifting heavy objects, bend with your knees bent, wear flat shoes, and always sit with your back well supported.

Bleeding gums Hormonal changes can cause a build-up of plaque on your teeth, which can lead to bleeding gums. It is important to pay special attention to oral hygiene and to avoid snacking on sweets and sugary drinks. Dental treatment is free while you are pregnant so have at least two check-ups during this time.

Cramp You may have a sudden sharp pain in your legs and feet, often at night. Try pulling your toes upwards towards your ankles and rub the affected muscles. Regular gentle exercise will help prevent cramp.

Constipation Some of the extra hormones produced in pregnancy can cause the intestines to relax and become less efficient. Eating plenty of fruit, vegetables and fibre, and drinking water will help.

Fainting You may feel faint if you stand for too long or get up too quickly. This happens because not enough blood is getting to your brain; if the oxygen level gets too low you may actually faint. Try to rise slowly from either sitting or lying positions and, if you are standing, sit down and lower your head towards your knees.

Piles Technically known as haemorrhoids, these are a form of varicose vein that appear around the back passage (anus). They can be very uncomfortable as they are itchy

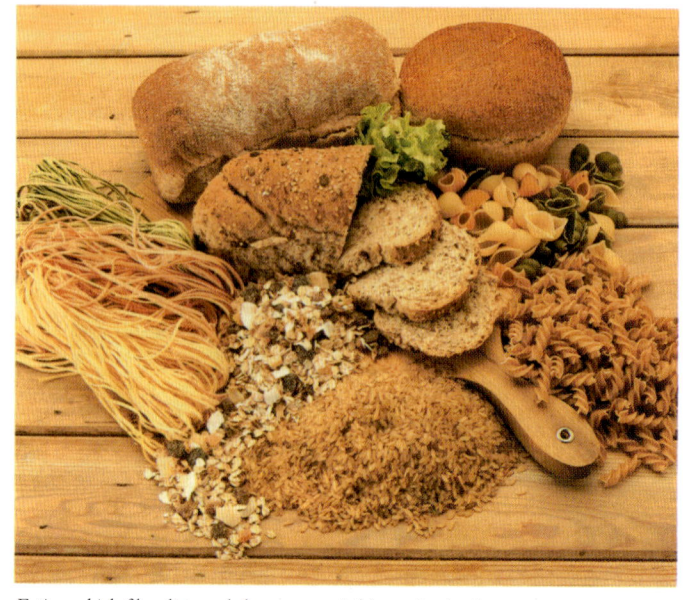

You and your body
Any sickness should start to fade and you will begin to feel less tired. You should start to think seriously about ante-natal classes because private ones can get booked up quickly. Contact your hospital or the National Childbirth Trust, or ask at your doctor's surgery about local classes.

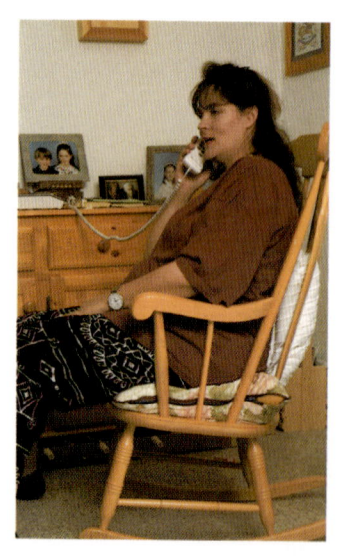

Your back is now more vulnerable, so support it with a cushion when you sit down.

Eating a high-fibre diet can help prevent painful constipation in pregnancy.

Week 11: Common Discomforts

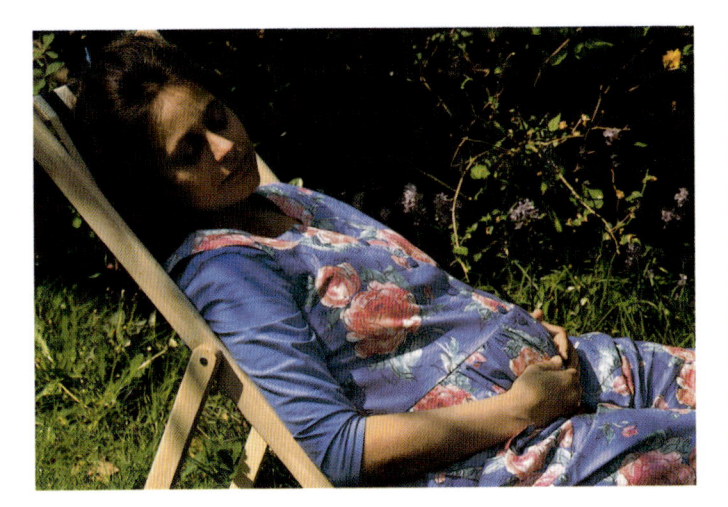

Your growing baby

Most of the major organs are formed, so the most vulnerable time will be over by the end of this week. The fetus is now relatively safe from any congenital abnormalities and infections, excepting rubella.

The external genitals have formed, along with either ovaries or testicles. The heart is now pumping blood to all the major organs of the body. The fetus weighs around 10 g/½ oz and is now about 5.5 cm/2⅛ in long.

Although you may now be feeling less tired than in the early weeks, you should still rest as much as you can.

and may even bleed slightly. If left untreated they can become prolapsed, which means they protrude through the anus, causing a good deal of pain. Eating high-fibre foods will keep your stools soft so that you don't have to strain, which puts pressure on piles. An ice pack wrapped in a soft cloth, or a witch hazel compress, will bring relief, or you can buy a specially formulated haemorrhoid preparation from the pharmacist. Piles usually disappear within a couple of weeks of the birth.

Vaginal discharge An increase in vaginal discharge during pregnancy is quite normal as long as the discharge is clear and white. If it becomes coloured, smells, or makes you itchy, you may have developed an infection, such as thrush, which will need treatment.

Take some gentle, regular exercise with your partner as this will help to prevent cramps and keep you feeling fit.

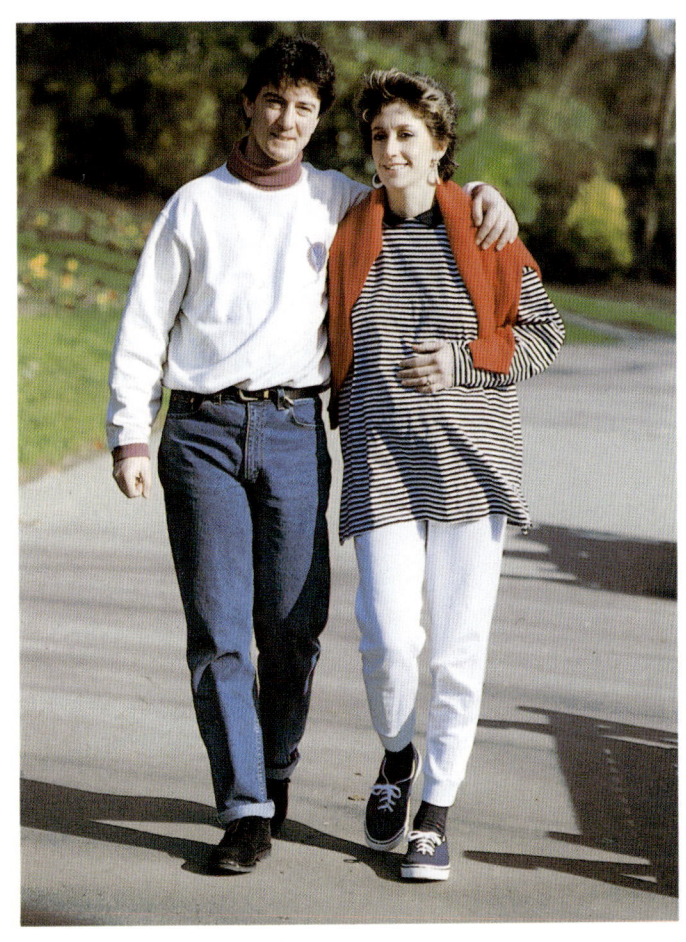

WEEK 12: HEALTHY EATING

The fetus gets all the nourishment it needs to grow from what you eat, so it is important to maintain a good diet throughout pregnancy. To achieve a healthy balanced diet you need to eat foods containing reasonable amounts of starchy carbohydrate, protein, fat, minerals, and vitamins each day. Starchy carbohydrates are found in bread, cereals, pasta, rice, and potatoes; they provide energy, vitamins, minerals, and fibre. Meat, fish, eggs, nuts, beans, peas, and lentils supply protein and minerals. Milk and dairy products such as hard cheese and yogurt will give you protein, vitamins, and calcium. Fresh fruit and vegetables and well-washed salads are good sources of minerals and vitamins. Folic acid can be found, with other vitamins, in green leafy vegetables, fruit, nuts, bread, and rice.

If you are a vegetarian, you will need to increase your milk intake to at least 600 ml/1 pint a day of either pasteurized milk or fortified soya milk, or the equivalent in cheese, yogurt, and dairy products.

Vegans will need to discuss their diet with a qualified dietitian as they could be deficient in calcium, iron, and vitamin B_{12}, which is found in foods of animal origin. Try to avoid eating sugary snacks and fizzy drinks and keep "junk" foods down to a minimum. Cut down on your caffeine intake from drinks like tea, coffee, chocolate and cola; try drinking bottled water and diluted fruit juices as alternatives.

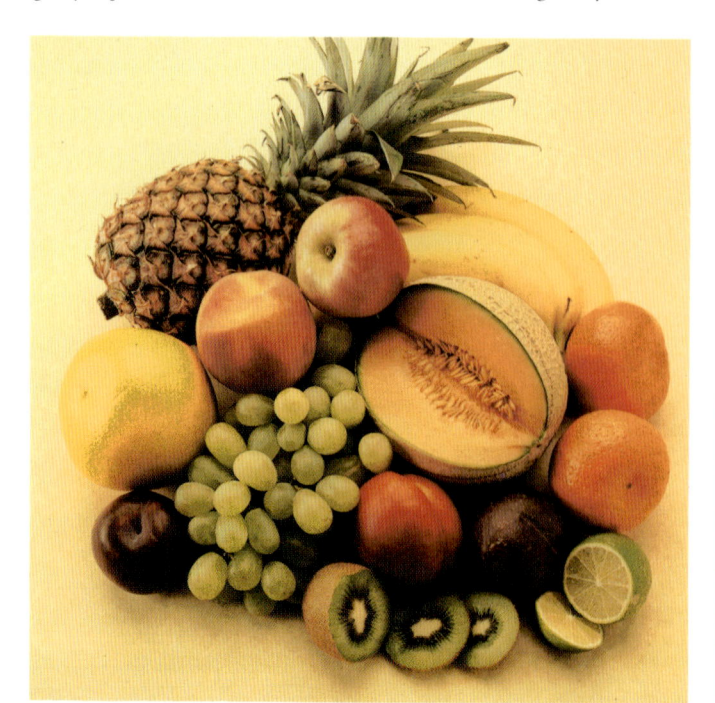

You and your body

You can expect to put on about one-quarter of your pregnancy weight between now and week 20. You may be beginning to feel more energetic and generally better than during the past few weeks. You should consider telling your employer at this time that you are pregnant.

Meanwhile, look at your lifestyle and be sure that your diet includes a sensible range of foods – for you and the unborn baby.

Eat plenty of fruit when pregnant as it is a good source of minerals and vitamins.

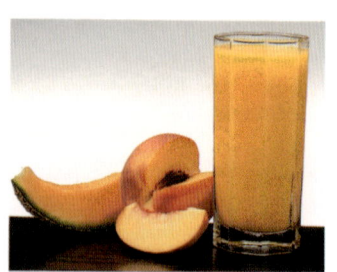

Cut down on your caffeine levels and drink more diluted fruit juices.

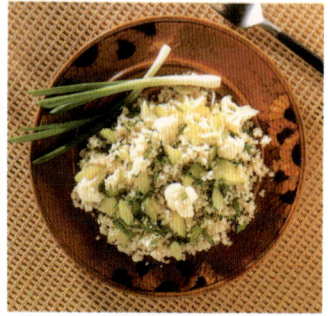

A grain salad will give you plenty of fibre.

WEEK 12: HEALTHY EATING

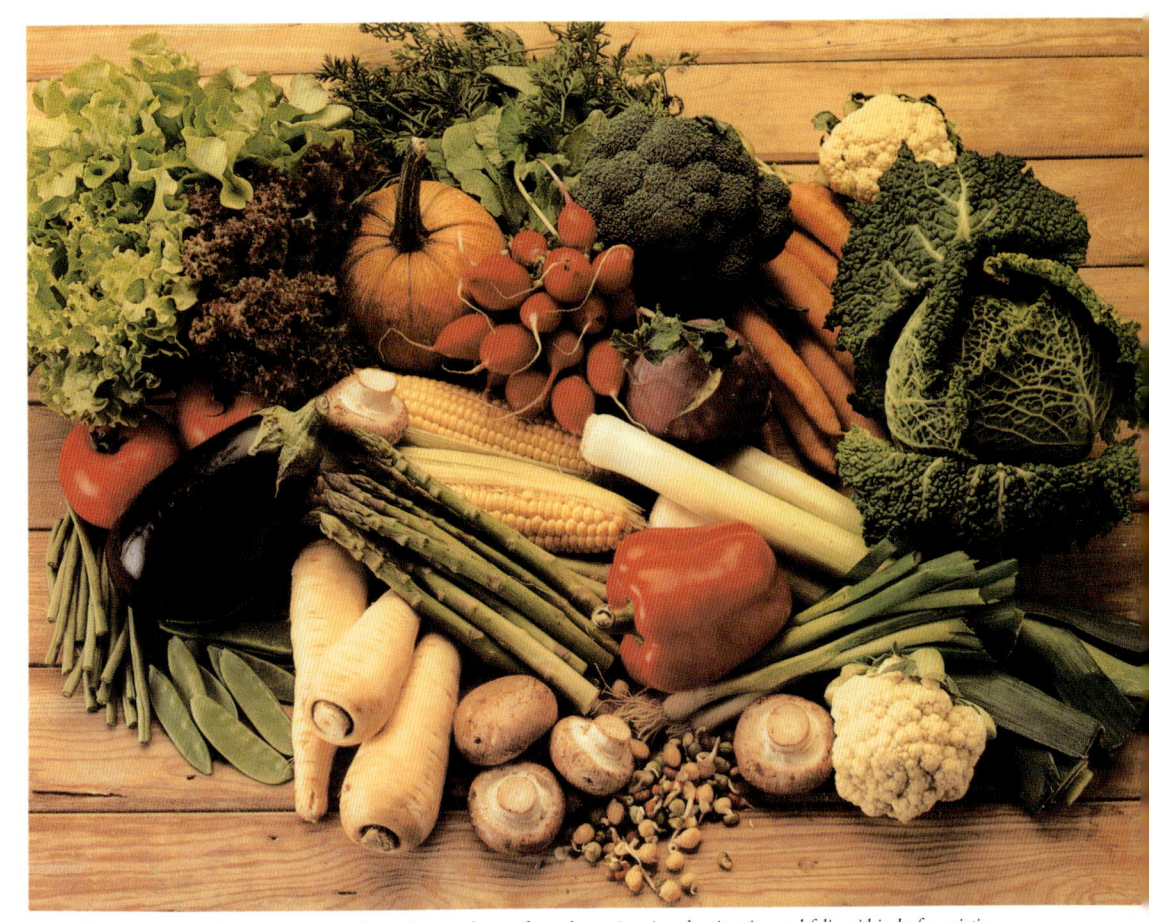

Vegetables are important in your pregnancy diet as they are low in fat and contain minerals, vitamins and folic acid in leafy varieties.

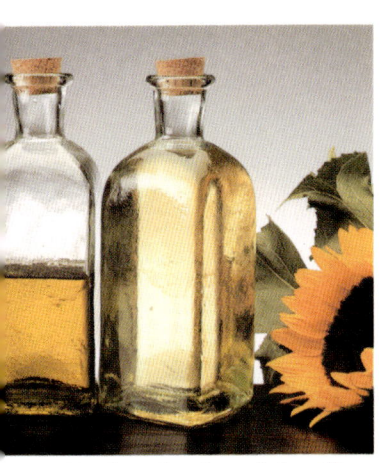

Use olive and sunflower oils for cooking.

YOUR WEIGHT

Although you need extra energy during pregnancy to meet the needs of the developing fetus, and to store fat ready for breast-feeding later, you are not likely to need special energy foods. If you were an acceptable weight for your build before pregnancy, the only extra calories you should need are during the last three months when you eat around 200 extra calories a day. However, if you were overweight or underweight your weight gain will need monitoring, and a special diet may be necessary. Ask a professional for advice.

Your growing baby

The fetus's heart is beating at between 110 and 160 times a minute and its chest is beginning to rise and fall as it practises future breathing movements. Features are becoming more clearly defined and fingers and toes are now fully formed, with tiny nails beginning to grow. The fetus can suck its thumb and it swallows amniotic fluid and passes it back as urine. The amniotic fluid is completely replaced every 24 hours. The fetus is now about 6.5 cm/2½ in long and weighs 20 g/¾ oz.

WEEK 13: THE HEALTH PROFESSIONALS

You and your body
Your uterus is enlarging at a noticeable rate and you will be able to see the first signs of a visible bump. Your nipples have become darker and the blue veins in your breasts are a lot more obvious.

Now that you are at the end of the first trimester and your pregnancy is a visible state, you should start to familiarize yourself with some of the professionals with whom you will regularly be interacting.

During pregnancy, and after the birth, a number of different people will be involved in your care. How many you see will depend on where you are having your baby and the kind of ante-natal care that is being offered. The type of professionals involved in your ante-natal and post-natal care will be the same wherever you are having your baby.

Midwife Your midwife has been trained to be an expert in pregnancy and she will care for you from the time your pregnancy is confirmed until after the birth of your baby. She will be able to give you physical and psychological support and to help with any medical problems that arise during this time.

Building up a relationship with you and your family is an essential part of the midwife's job, so it is important for you to establish contact with her as soon after your pregnancy is confirmed as possible. Your midwife will usually be found at your local health centre or your doctor's surgery, although it may also be possible to contact her direct through the Supervisor of Midwives at your local maternity unit.

Your midwife will be able to help you make an informed choice about your right to have your baby where and how you wish. She will advise you on the most appropriate care for your needs and, if specialist help is required, she will know the right person to contact. The midwife will continue to look after you and your family until she hands over your care to a health visitor at between 10 and 28 days after the birth.

Health visitor The health visitor is a fully-qualified nurse who has had extra training in caring for people in the community. Her role is to help families, especially those with very young children. Your health visitor will visit you at home sometime after your baby is 10 days old. She will give you information about feeding, as well as general health and safety, and can offer advice and give support if you have any worries about your baby or if you yourself have any problems.

The health visitor will give you a telephone number where she can be contacted if you need help. You can arrange to see her at home, or at the child health clinic, health centre, or doctor's surgery.

General practitioner Your GP will probably have confirmed your pregnancy and will be able to help you plan your ante-natal care. He or she may be responsible for all or part of your ante-natal care and will work closely with your midwife. If you are having a home birth, your GP may be involved in your baby's delivery, together with your midwife. If you are going to have a hospital birth

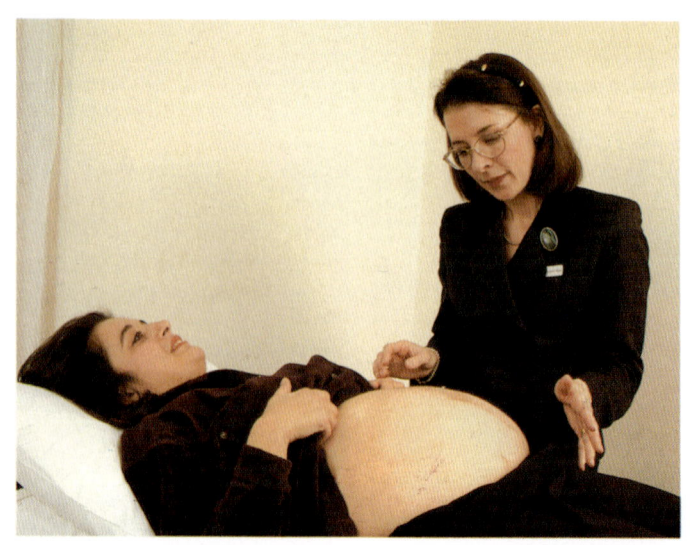

As your pregnancy progresses you may be examined by an obstetrician who specializes in birth and child care. She will advise on your baby's development and discuss any problems.

Week 13: The Health Professionals

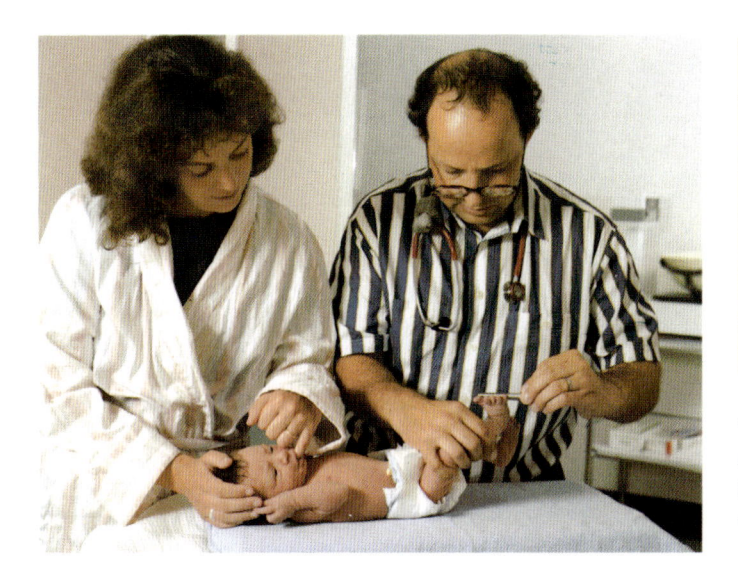

Your growing baby
The fetus is now 7.5 cm/3 in long and weighs 30 g/1½ oz. The bone marrow, liver, and spleen have now taken over production of blood cells. The bones are developing and the teeth are in place. The fetus may already be practising lip movements to develop the muscles needed for the sucking reflex after the birth.

The pediatrician will perform several checks on your baby after birth. Here he is checking that the newborn's foot reflex works correctly.

your GP should come and visit you and your baby soon after you get back home.

You need to register your baby with the GP as soon after the birth as possible. You can contact your GP at any time if either you or your baby are ill. Your doctor may have an arrangement where young babies are seen without making an appointment, possibly at the beginning or end of the surgery, or it may be possible to obtain some advice over the phone. Your GP may hold a clinic at the surgery, and will normally work closely with the health visitors in your area.

Obstetrician This is a doctor who specializes in the care of women throughout their pregnancy and subsequent childbirth. If you are having a delivery in a hospital, the consultant you are under will be an obstetrician who is part of a special medical team.

Pediatrician This is a doctor who specializes in caring for babies and children. Your baby will be checked by a pediatrician after the birth.

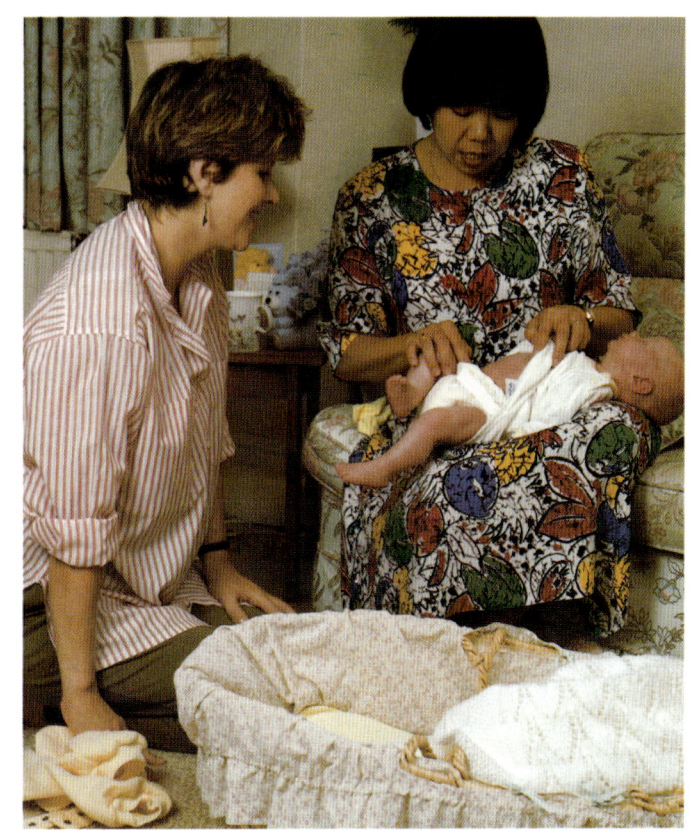

Your health visitor will visit you after your baby's birth and check that the navel is healing.

THE SECOND TRIMESTER

WEEK 14: SEX DURING PREGNANCY

To be able to enjoy sex it is important to know that making love cannot harm the developing fetus. It is well protected in the uterus by the amniotic fluid and membranes, and the uterus itself is sealed with a plug of mucus, which stays in place until just before the birth. Even deep penetration is safe, but it should of course be gentle so that it doesn't cause discomfort.

Many women find that the middle months of pregnancy are a sensual and even erotic time. Physical changes, such as the increase in the size of your breasts, can actually serve to heighten your interest in sex, which in turn leads to an increase in sexual pleasure. Your genitals may also appear bigger and the pressure from the growing baby can actually make them more responsive. Some women find that they experience orgasm for the first time during pregnancy, while others come to orgasm much more quickly.

Experiencing orgasm is perfectly safe, in fact it can be considered to be beneficial since the uterus often remains hard and firm for several minutes afterwards. This is similar in effect to the Braxton Hicks, or practice contractions you experience towards the end of your pregnancy that prepare the uterus for the birth of your baby.

You may of course find that you feel a lessening of desire during pregnancy, or even a complete loss of interest in sex. These feelings are not uncommon, but they can cause unnecessary stress between you and your partner if they are not brought out into the open and discussed.

You and your body

You are now beginning the second trimester when you should start experiencing what is known as mid-pregnancy bloom. You will be feeling better about everything; if your sex drive has diminished over the last few months it will probably return and sex may be better than ever.

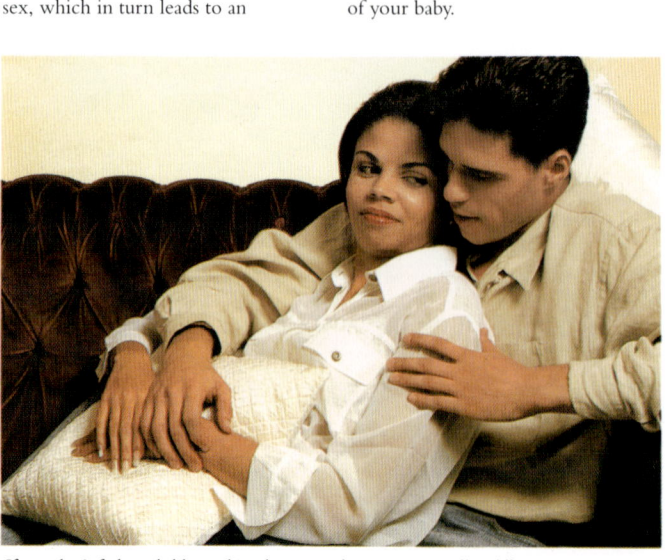

If you don't feel much like making love in early pregnancy, still cuddle your partner and show him lots of affection.

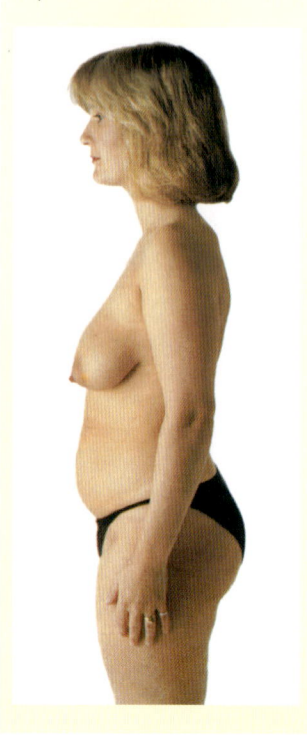

Week 14: Sex During Pregnancy

Your partner may feel that he is being rejected, so it is important to find alternative ways of giving each other love and reassurance.

Different ways to make love

It is important that you and your partner show each other physical affection during pregnancy, but this does not always have to involve sexual intercourse. You may find as your pregnancy progresses that you want lots of cuddles and other signs of affection from your partner without actually having sex. Men often find this hard to understand as they tend to link such physical contact with intercourse. Explain to your partner how you feel so that together you can find other ways of expressing your love for each other.

Try experimenting with different forms of sex play that don't necessarily end in penetration, so that you can still make love even if you don't feel like intercourse. Take time to

Your growing baby
The fetus is beginning to look human as the chin, forehead, and nose become more clearly defined. It can now turn its head and even wrinkle its brow. The fetus may even respond to external stimulus by actually moving away when the doctor or midwife feels your abdomen. The fetus is now 9 cm/3½ in long and weighs about 60 g/2 oz.

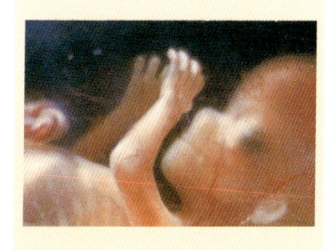

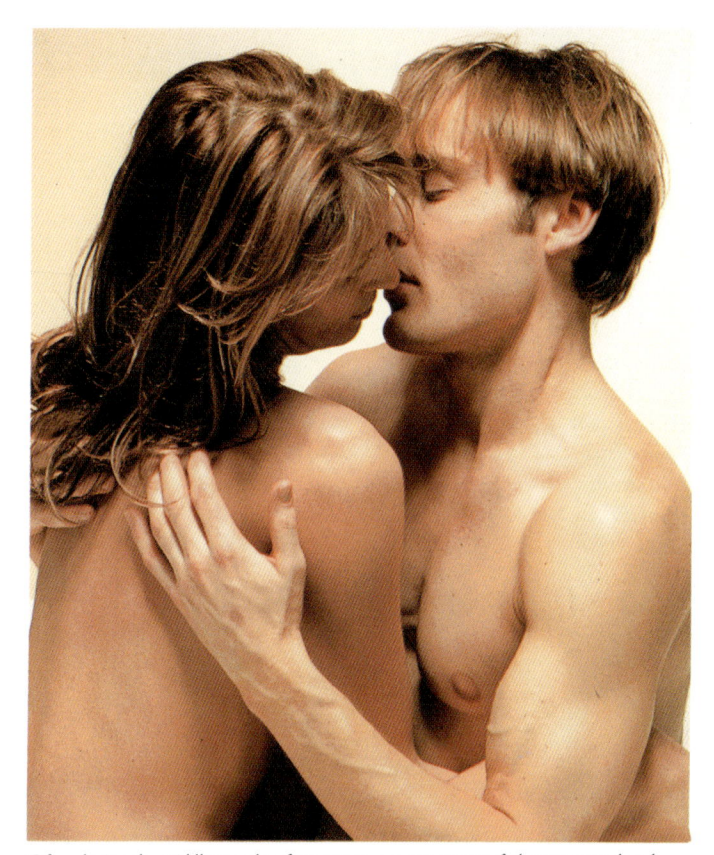

Often during the middle months of pregnancy, you can start to feel more sensual and show renewed interest in sex.

find out what you both enjoy and don't be afraid to tell your partner what you do and don't like.

Stroking, massage, mutual masturbation, and oral sex are some alternative ways of making love which you can both enjoy and which may at times be more appropriate than full intercourse.

As you grow larger you'll find some positions for lovemaking more comfortable than others. Experiment with positions which keep your partner's weight off you.

Using sex to induce labour

Sex can sometimes be a way of inducing labour. Your partner's semen contains a hormone called prostaglandin, which will help to soften the cervix in preparation for birth. Lovemaking will also stimulate the cells in the cervix to secrete their own prostaglandins; this too may help bring labour on.

Breast stimulation in late pregnancy sometimes produces quite strong contractions which are thought to help prepare the way for labour by softening and drawing up the cervix. It has been discovered that stimulating nipples can reactivate a labour that has halted – something that your partner might like to remember.

WEEK 15: HEALTH AND SAFETY

You may hear about risks during pregnancy. Some are valid, others are based on misinformation.

If you work with dangerous substances such as chemicals or in a job which requires you to do heavy lifting, you could be risking your health and the health of your child. Your employer must offer you an alternative job if yours is a recognized risk. If you are concerned about risks at work talk to your doctor, your employer, or union representative.

A common concern among working women is that sitting all day in front of a VDU screen such as a computer terminal or word processor will harm the developing fetus. The most recent research shows no evidence of this being a risk, but you may need to have your microwave checked out for any minor radiation leaks, although with modern equipment these are very unlikely.

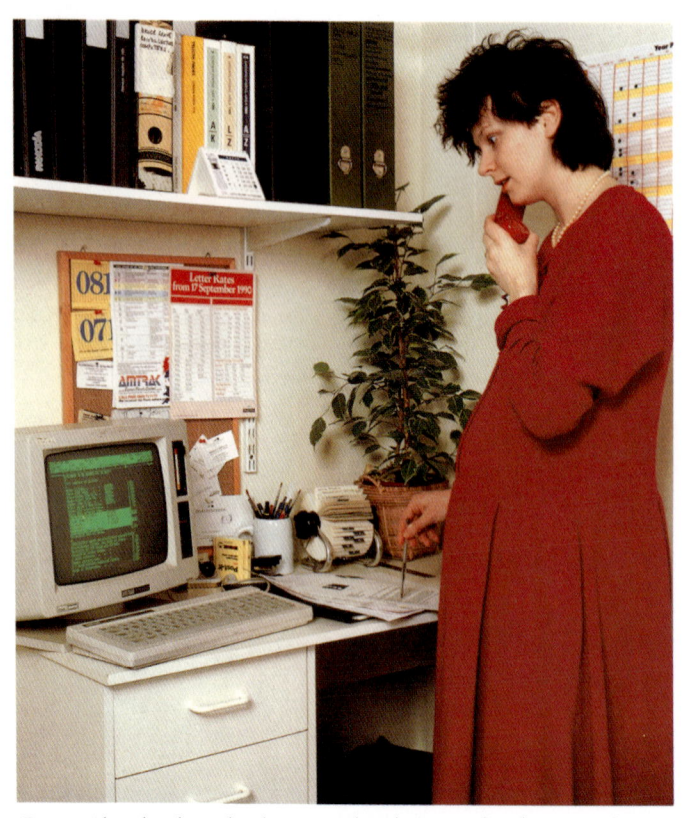

Recent evidence has shown that there is no risk to the growing fetus for women who regularly use computer terminals. However, move around often to minimize backache.

You and your body
Your heart has enlarged to cope with the increased amount of blood circulating in your body and the fetus's need for oxygen, and has increased its output by 20 per cent. You will be feeling more energetic than before and now is a good time to have a holiday before the birth.

HEALTH HAZARDS
While you are pregnant you should avoid eating unpasteurized milk and products made with unpasteurized milk; pâté made from meat, fish, or vegetables; soft and blue vein cheeses; soft-whip ice cream; pre-cooked poultry and cook-chill meals; and prepared salads (unless washed thoroughly) because of the risk of listeria.

Listeria monocytogenes is the bacterium which causes listeriosis in humans and animals. Animals that carry the bacterium are likely to infect the milk they produce and the meat that is produced from them. The bacterium is usually destroyed during the pasteurization of milk and milk products. However, if food is contaminated and then refrigerated the bacteria will continue to multiply. Listeriosis can also be spread through direct contact with animals that are infected.

Toxoplasmosis is a disease that occurs in both humans and animals. It can be extremely dangerous if it is contracted during pregnancy because it may cause miscarriage or severe fetal abnormality. The disease is spread to humans by eating undercooked or raw meat and through coming into contact with cat faeces. The infection can also be caught from sheep at lambing time. As it is

Week 15: Health and Safety

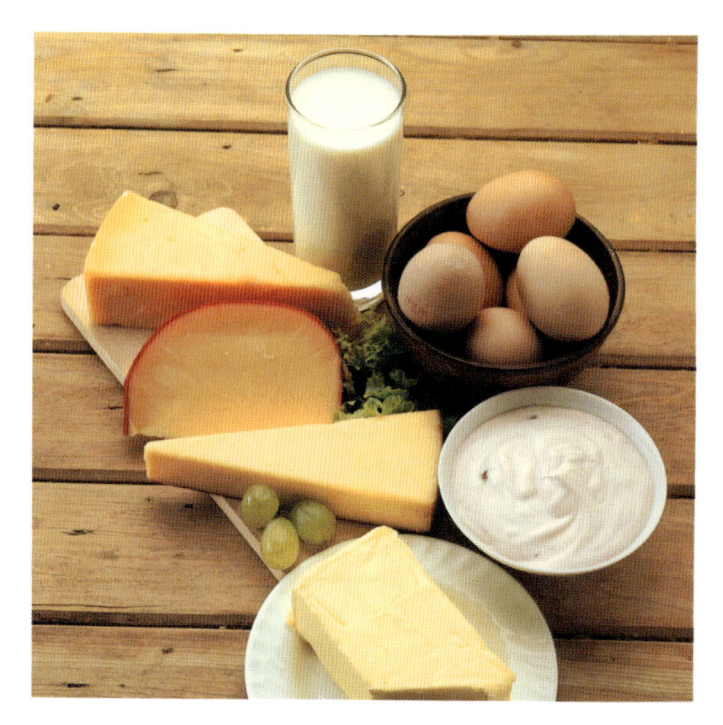

Your growing baby

The fetal skeleton is developing and its legs are now longer than its arms. The hair on its head is becoming thicker and it has eyelashes as well as eyebrows. The fetus can probably hear now and the amniotic fluid makes an excellent sound conductor, so it will be able to hear your stomach rumbling and your heart beating as well as the sound of your voice. The fetus is 12 cm/4¾ in long and now weighs 100 g/3½ oz.

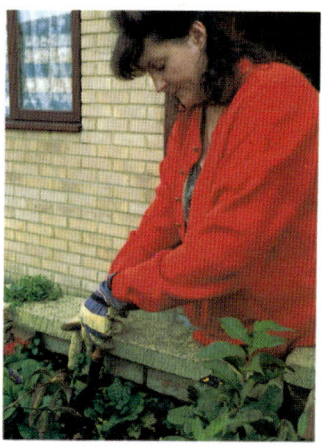

quite possible to have the disease without knowing it, you should have a blood test to find out whether or not you have immunity. If you are immune, you definitely cannot infect your baby.

If you find that you are not immune, you should take a number of precautions during pregnancy. Avoid any meat that has not been cooked thoroughly and wash your hands, cooking utensils, and surfaces after preparing raw meat. Wash fruit and vegetables to remove all traces of soil. Avoid unpasteurized goats' milk and goats' milk products. Finally, wear rubber gloves when gardening and wash your hands afterwards. Cover your children's sand boxes in the garden to prevent any cats from using them as litter trays. Always wear rubber gloves when handling cat litter, and wash your hands and the gloves afterwards.

Above: Hard cheeses are safe to eat in pregnancy. However, make sure you only eat hard-boiled eggs and drink pasteurized milk to avoid Listeria monocytogenes. *Right: Always wear some gloves when gardening during pregnancy as toxoplasmosis can be caught from cat faeces.*

Food safety

Avoid putting yourself at risk during pregnancy by taking the following precautions with food.
- Wash all fruit, vegetables, and salads, including any pre-packed salads, thoroughly.
- Don't eat raw or undercooked meat.
- Eggs must be well cooked and all dairy products should be pasteurized.
- Avoid eating any soft, imported cheeses such as Brie and Camembert, blue-vein cheeses, and those that are made from goats' and sheep's milk because of the risk of listeria.
- Don't eat liver and liver products, such as pâté and liver sausage. They contain high levels of vitamin A, which is toxic in excess amounts.
- Avoid cook-chill meals and shellfish.
- Keep your fridge below 5°C/41°F and don't refreeze any previously frozen foods.
- Pay special attention to hygiene in the kitchen.
- Don't eat food that is past its "sell by" or "best before" date.

WEEK 16: SCANS/TWINS

At around 16 weeks you will probably be offered an ultrasound scan so that you can see your baby for the first time. A scan can be carried out at any stage of pregnancy, but is usually offered between 16 and 20 weeks (although a dating scan may be offered as early as ten weeks).

The procedure is completely painless. High-density sound waves are used to create a picture of your baby in the uterus, and you will be able to see this on a screen. The best pictures are obtained when you have a full bladder so you will be asked to drink a lot of fluid beforehand. You lie on a couch and your stomach is lubricated so that the person performing the scan can pull the scanner smoothly across it. The picture that appears on the screen may not be clear, so ask the radiographer to explain the images to you, if you are unsure of what you are seeing.

The fetus's age can be determined from a scan; it also shows up most abnormalities of the head and spine that may have occurred and will detect the presence of twins. The exact position of the placenta and the fetus can be seen, so if there are any problems, for example when the placenta is situated very low down, extra care will be taken throughout your pregnancy.

TWINS

There is about a one in 80 chance that you and your partner will conceive twins. However, you are more likely to give birth to twins if you have a history of them in your, or your partner's, family.

Identical twins come from one egg which, once fertilized, then splits into two separate cells. Each of the cells then grows into a separate fetus, but they usually share the same placenta. Because identical twins originally came from the same cells they are always the same sex and look like each other.

Non-identical twins, also known as fraternal twins, are the result of two eggs being fertilized by two different sperm at the same time. Each fetus has its own placenta and the sexes of the babies may differ.

Fraternal twins usually don't look any more alike than brothers and sisters who are born years apart.

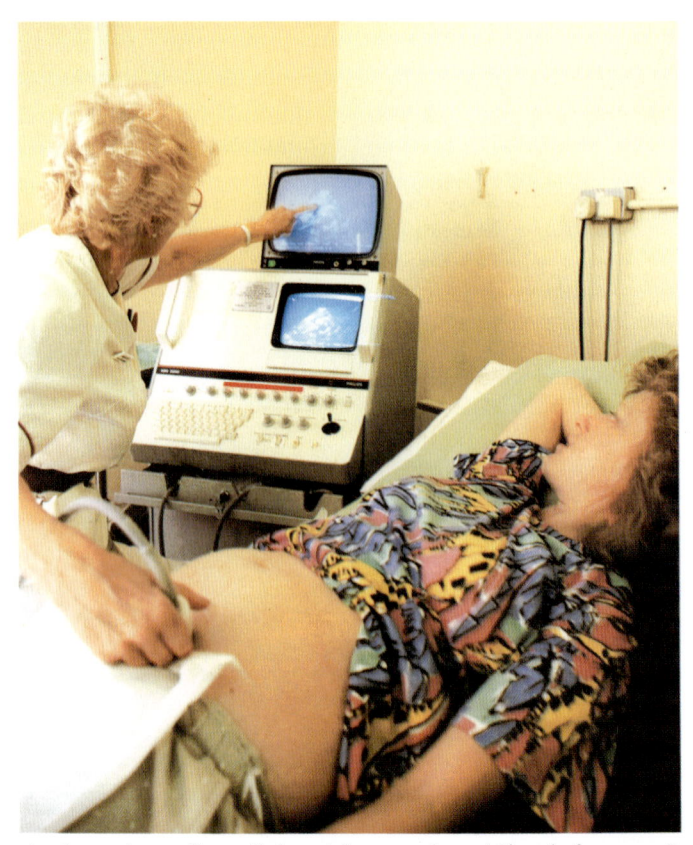

You and your body

You may feel your baby's first movements around this time. These early movements are like a fluttering, bubbling sensation. You may notice the beginning of *Linea nigra*, a dark line which appears down the centre of your abdomen. This will disappear after the birth.

An ultrasound scan will normally be carried out around your 16th week of pregnancy. It will show up any abnormalities in your baby and also indicate the presence of twins.

WEEK 16: SCANS/TWINS

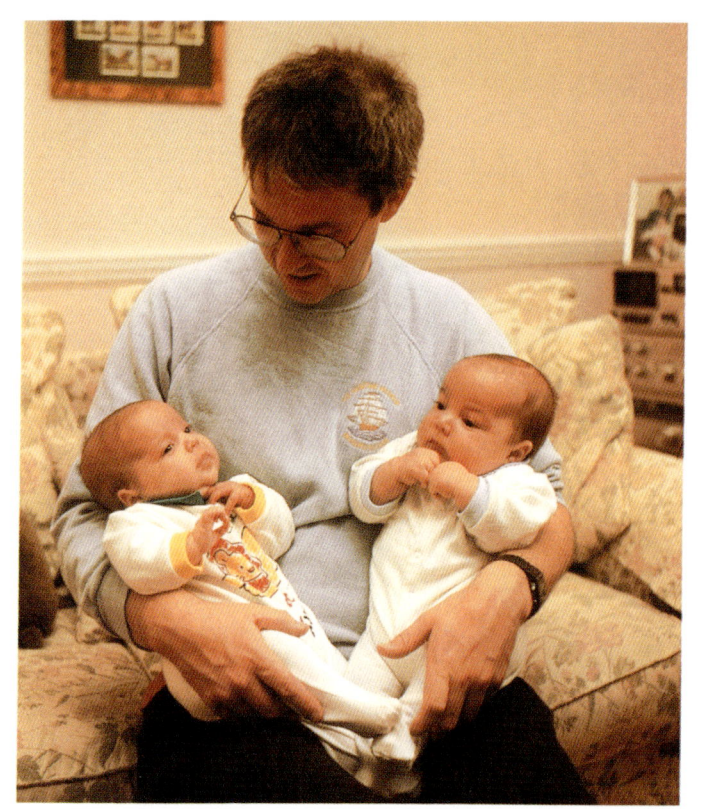

Your growing baby

The fetus will be moving around frequently now, although you may have only just started to feel these movements. The body will become covered in a fine downy hair called lanugo, which is thought to maintain the right body temperature. It is possible to tell a baby's sex now through an ultrasound scan. The fetus is 16 cm/6¼ in long and weighs 135 g/5 oz.

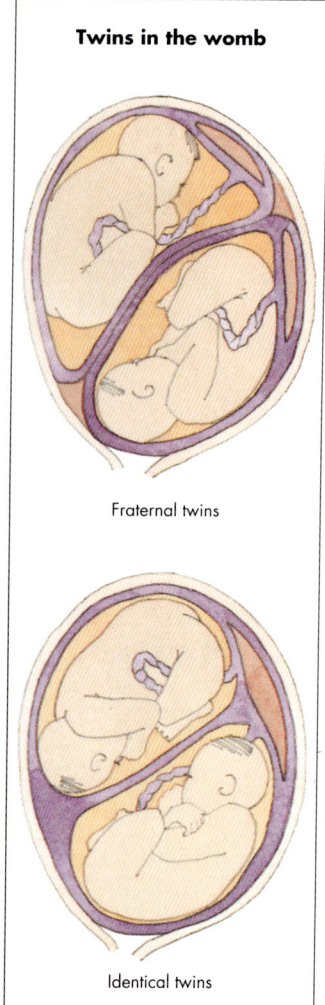

The arrival of twins can come as rather a shock. Get your partner to help as much as he can and you will soon find that you both start bonding with them.

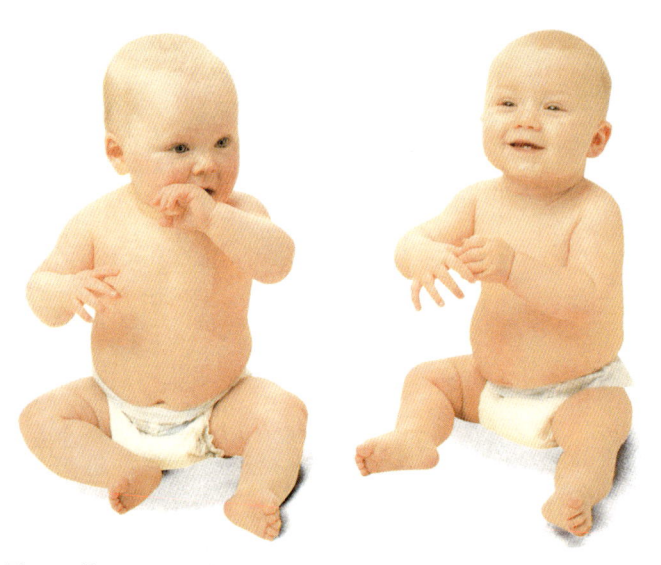

Twins in the womb

Fraternal twins

Identical twins

The joy of having twins is that as they grow up they will learn to play with each other.

WEEK 17: YOUR PREGNANCY WARDROBE

You will find that loose ordinary clothes, in a bigger size if necessary, will see you through most of your pregnancy. A few basic garments that are interchangeable will help you achieve a variety of looks. Buy skirts and trousers with elasticated waists, baggy shirts, and big T-shirts in natural fibres such as cotton. Choose underwear with some cotton content for softness and absorbency and maternity tights or stockings to give your legs support. As your breasts are likely to increase in size rapidly during the early months of pregnancy, it makes sense to buy a well-fitting support bra early. This will prevent your breasts sagging which will help them to return to their normal shape once the baby is born.

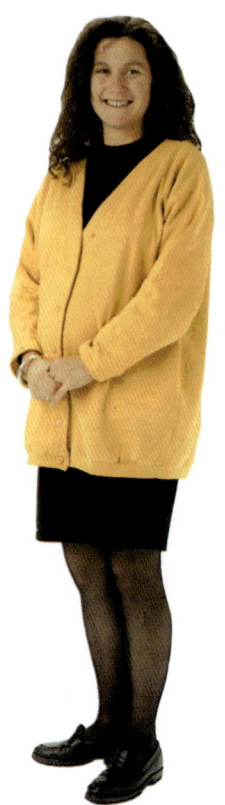

A baggy cardigan worn over a skirt with an elasticated waist helps conceal your bump.

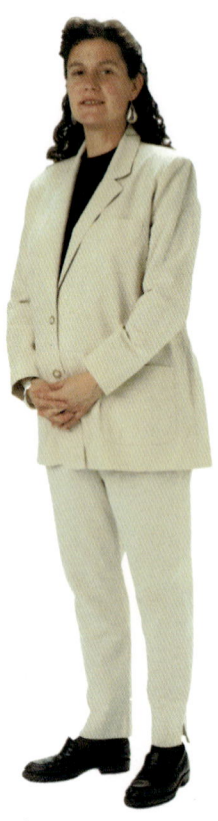

A loose-fitting trouser suit with a long jacket can look and feel good in pregnancy.

You and your body
Your waistline will have completely disappeared and you may have begun to develop stretch marks. Bleeding gums may be a problem, so if you haven't had a dental check-up now is the time to go. If you work, you should start thinking about when you intend to leave and whether you will want to return.

Your growing baby
All your baby's limbs are now fully formed as well as the skin and muscle. Its taste buds are beginning to develop so that it will be able to distinguish sweet from non-sweetened fluid. The fetus is now about 18 cm/7 in long and weighs around 185 g/6½ oz.

Maternity rights and benefits
Once your pregnancy is confirmed, you should make enquiries about your maternity rights and benefits. You will probably be entitled to some financial and/or medical benefits from the government. If you work you may qualify for statutory maternity pay from your employer. This may be in the form of a weekly allowance which is paid by your employer. You are entitled to take time off work to attend ante-natal clinics and parentcraft classes, so you will need to let your employer know that you are pregnant before your booking-in visit. Your midwife or health visitor will be able to give you help or advice if you are unsure of what to do.

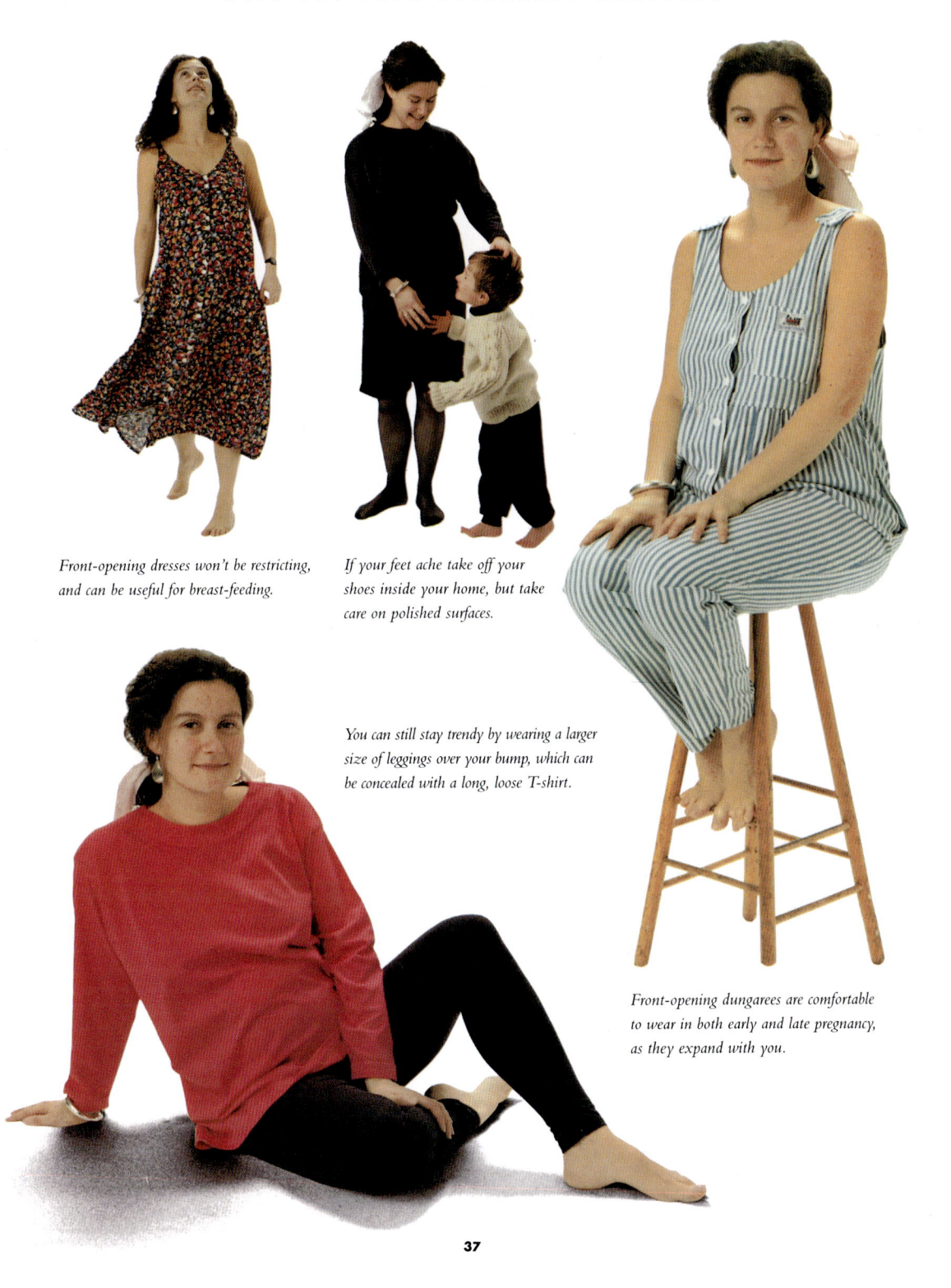

WEEK 17: YOUR PREGNANCY WARDROBE

Front-opening dresses won't be restricting, and can be useful for breast-feeding.

If your feet ache take off your shoes inside your home, but take care on polished surfaces.

You can still stay trendy by wearing a larger size of leggings over your bump, which can be concealed with a long, loose T-shirt.

Front-opening dungarees are comfortable to wear in both early and late pregnancy, as they expand with you.

WEEK 18: LOOKING YOUR BEST

You may find that your hair behaves in a rather unpredictable way while you are pregnant. Hormone changes mean that your hair may appear thicker than usual, or in some women the opposite happens and the hair loss increases so that the hair looks thinner. Dry hair may become even drier and oily hair more greasy. Whichever condition applies to you, just wash your hair using a mild shampoo. If your hair tends to be very dry, use a good conditioner after every wash and, if possible, allow it to dry naturally rather than using a hair dryer.

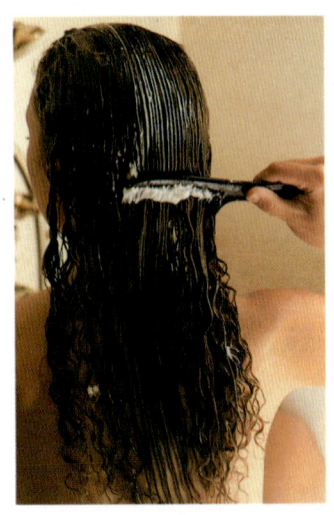

Dry hair will need extra conditioning during your pregnancy because it becomes drier as your hormones change.

Pregnancy hormones can affect the colour and texture of your skin. Uneven patches appear and dark-skinned people may even get a but-

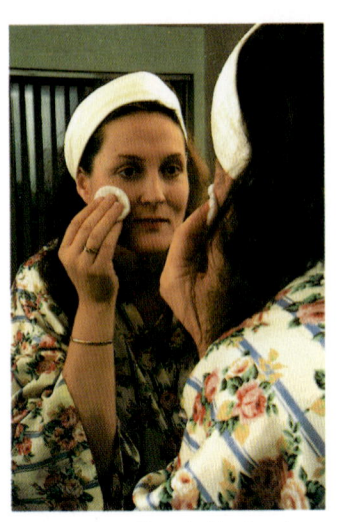

Try using hypoallergenic skin-cleansing products on your skin as it will be particularly sensitive at this time.

terfly-shaped patch of pigmentation across the face which is known as "the mask of pregnancy" Concealing foundation will help hide these marks and a UVA sun screen will prevent any further increase in pigmentation. Pregnancy "bloom", which is caused by an increase in the tiny blood vessels under the surface of the skin, can be toned down with green cream or powder. It is a good idea to use hypoallergenic skin-care products as your skin may be particularly sensitive at this time.

FLUID RETENTION

Your body retains more water than usual during pregnancy, so your hands and feet may become slightly swollen and you may find that your eyes get puffy and your face looks fuller. The best solution is to get as much rest as possible, sitting with your feet higher than your heart, as this will help reduce the swelling in your feet and ankles. While you are resting, place some cottonwool pads soaked in witch hazel, or slices of cucumber, on your eyes. This will soothe them and reduce any puffiness. You can disguise a fuller face by applying blusher below the cheekbones and blending a darker shade of foundation along your jawline. Alternatively, you can draw attention away from your face by wearing a colourful scarf or a chunky necklace round your neck.

Try not to be too critical of your looks; many other people will consider that this new, softer look to your appearance makes you seem younger and healthier.

You and your body
You should be able to feel the fetal movements quite clearly now. Your nose may become blocked as pregnancy causes the membranes inside the nasal passages to swell. You may also notice an increase in vaginal discharge. You will find that there are several physical changes besides the predictable weight gain.

Your growing baby
The skin is still wrinkled because the fetus hasn't started to gain body fat and is very active. It is becoming aware of sounds outside the uterus and you may be able to feel it jumping at unexpected noises. The fetus is now around 21 cm/8½ in long and weighs about 235 g/8 oz.

Week 18: Looking Your Best

With extra care you can transform your face from looking tired and pale in pregnancy (left) to attractive and striking (right). A concealing foundation masks any pigmentation marks, mascara and soft eye shadows can highlight your eyes, and a stunning lipstick can emphasize your mouth.

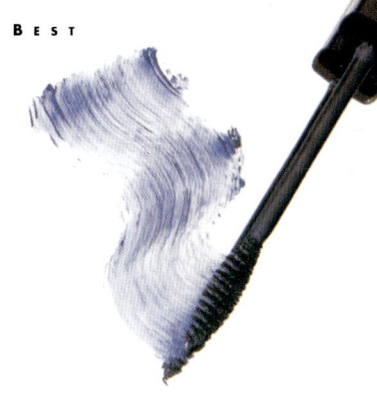

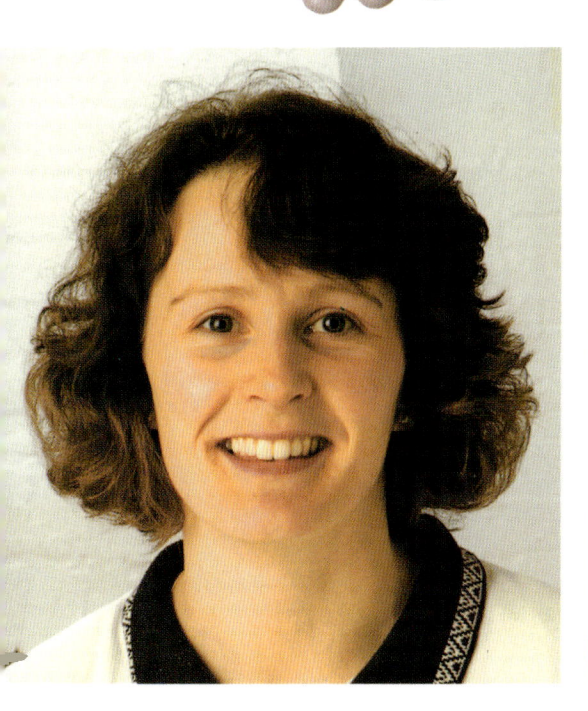

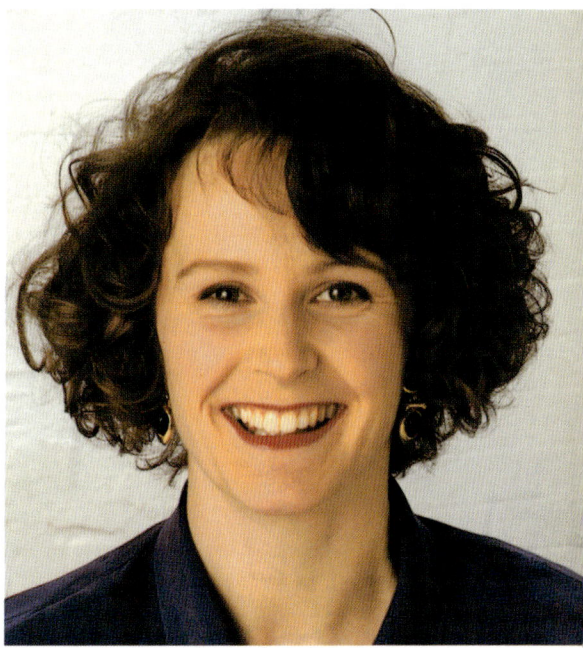

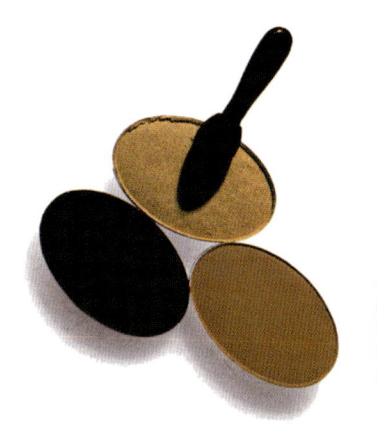

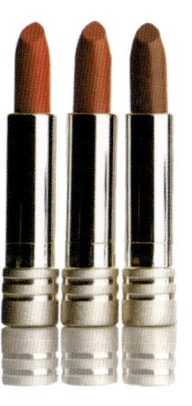

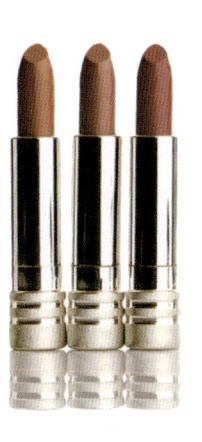

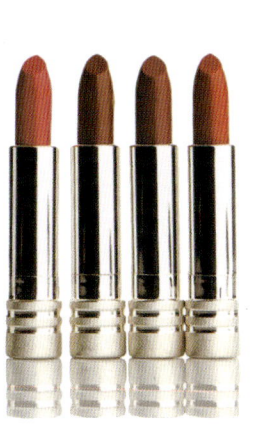

WEEK 19: EXERCISE

Regular, gentle exercise has an important part to play in keeping you fit during pregnancy and will help you get back into shape after the birth. Remember, if you ever feel faint, light-headed or breathless while you are exercising you must stop immediately. If you haven't been taking exercise, start swimming, or take up yoga or walking as they can all be done at a gentle, rhythmical pace which can be adapted to suit each stage of your pregnancy. If you find it easier to follow an exercise routine you can do at home, never include sit-ups or exercises that involve raising the legs when you are lying down as these could damage the abdominal muscles. It is important to stop and relax between exercises and to make sure that your breathing always remains at a controlled rate.

You and your body

You have started to put weight on your bottom, hips, and thighs as well as your abdomen. Tiny veins may start appearing on your face. These are very small broken blood vessels which are caused by circulation changes. They will disappear after the birth.

Toning your breasts

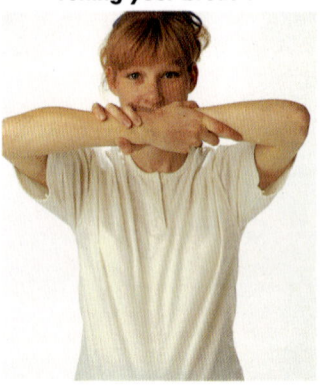

1 Hold arms at breast level with hands loosely clasping opposite arm. Tighten grip and hold briefly, then relax.

2 Still keeping your hands clasped, raise them to eye level and tighten your grip and hold, then relax.

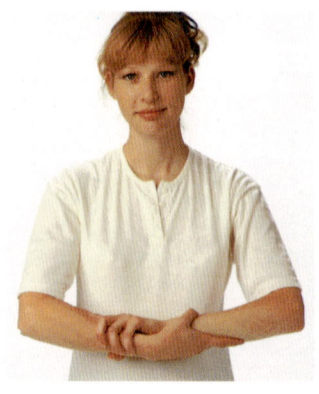

3 Lower your arms down to your waist, tighten and hold, then relax. Repeat this sequence several times.

Feet exercises

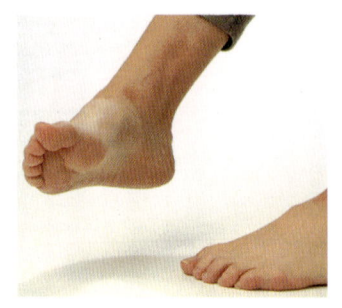

1 To loosen ankles, sit down with feet flat on the ground. Lift one foot at a time and circle ankle five times in both directions.

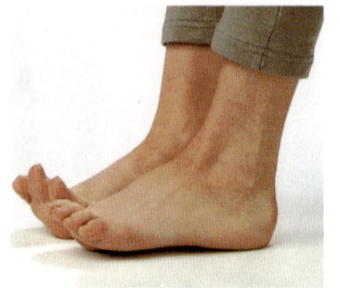

2 To tone the feet, place your feet flat on the floor. Now lift your toes up as far as you can and hold briefly, then relax.

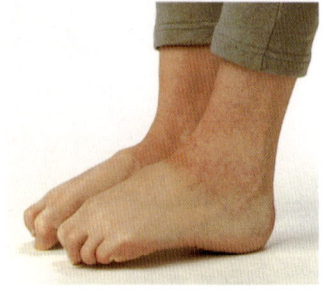

3 Now clench your toes hard, hold for a few seconds, then relax again. Repeat this technique, and Step 2, 10 times.

Week 19: Exercise

Taylor sitting and squatting exercises

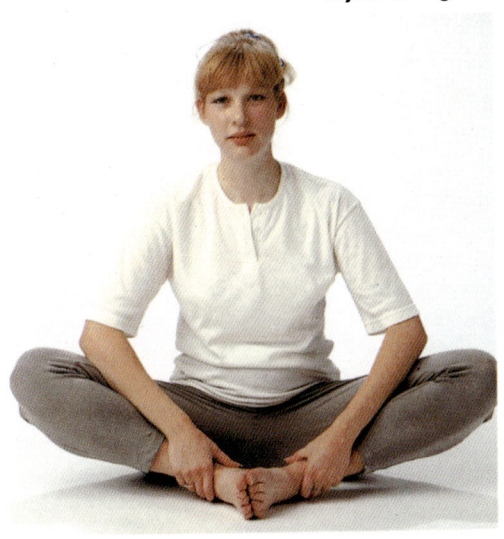

1 To loosen the groin and hips and stretch the inner thighs, sit with the soles of your feet together. Holding ankles, bring your pelvis and feet together by moving your hips towards your feet.

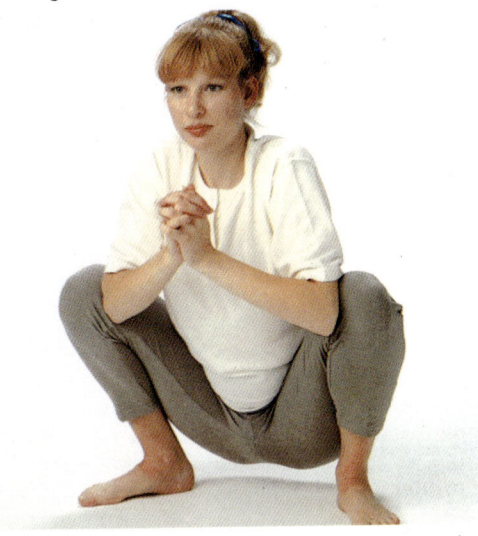

2 This is a good position for labour. Squat down keeping a straight back; try to put your heels down placing your weight evenly. Press your elbows against your thighs stretching the inner groin and thighs.

Tummy toning exercises

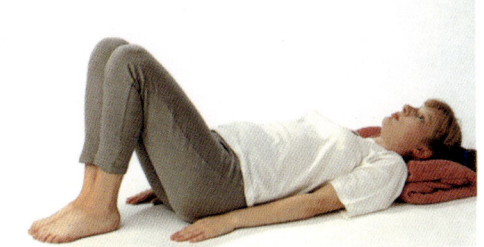

1 Put a folded towel or pillow under your head and lie with your knees bent and your feet flat on the floor. Press the small of your back down on the floor.

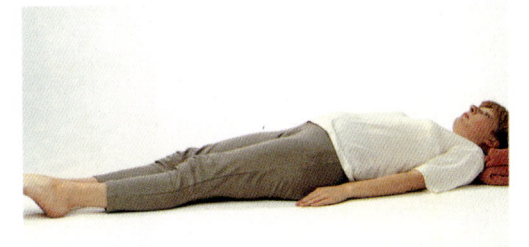

2 Slowly extend both your legs in front of you until they are both completely straight, but still keep your back pressed well down onto the floor.

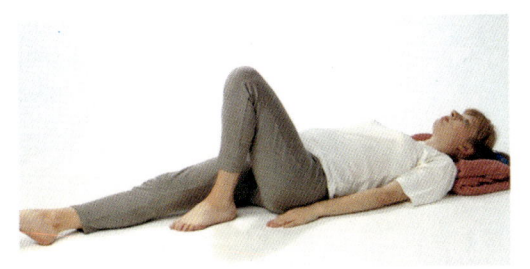

3 Draw one knee up and then the other, without lifting your back off the floor. Relax your legs until straight; repeat five times.

Your growing baby

The fetus is starting to put on weight and its rapid rate of growth has begun to slow down. The milk teeth have developed in the gums and the buds for the permanent teeth are beginning to form. The fetus is around 23 cm/9 in long and weighs about 285 g/10 oz.

WEEK 20: SKIN CARE/CRAVINGS

> **You and your body**
> Your uterus is enlarging quite rapidly now so that you look pregnant. Your navel may be flattened or pushed out and it will stay this way until after the birth. Heartburn may start to become a problem because the uterus is starting to push against your stomach.

Your breasts are likely to increase by as much as two bra sizes during pregnancy, so you will need to make sure that they are well supported so that they do not sag and become uncomfortable. Small bumps may appear in the skin around your nipples. These are sebaceous glands which secrete sebum, a fatty lubricant. As your pregnancy progresses, your nipples grow softer and gentle massage will help make them supple and ready for breast-feeding. Your breasts may leak a yellow fluid called colostrum, which will form a crust on the nipples. You will need to wash and dry them gently and thoroughly at least twice a day.

Your nails are made of protein and are affected by the hormonal changes taking place in your body. Usually they grow longer and stronger during pregnancy, but occasionally pregnancy will cause them to split and break. If this happens, keep them short and protect them by wearing gloves when you are doing rough jobs or when you immerse your hands in water.

If the elasticity of your skin becomes overstretched as you put on weight, you may develop stretch marks. These usually appear on the breasts, stomach, and the tops of the thighs as thin, reddish lines. There is little you can do to avoid them, but keeping your skin well moisturized, and being careful not to put on too much extra weight, will help minimize them. Stretch marks fade to thin silvery lines after the birth.

Varicose veins can be caused by pregnancy hormones or, later in pregnancy, by the uterus pressing down and obstructing the flow of blood from the legs to the heart. Although not serious, they can lead to aching or sore legs. Try to avoid standing for long periods and put your feet up whenever possible to ease any discomfort. Walking will help the blood flow; put on support tights or stockings when you get out of bed in the morning to give your legs more support. Varicose veins usually disappear soon after the birth.

Cravings

No one is sure why some pregnant women have cravings while others don't. Doctors disagree about them; some are sympathetic while others doubt that they actually exist. If you desire a certain food there is no reason why you shouldn't indulge yourself within reason, but make sure that you don't exclude other more nourishing foods as a result.

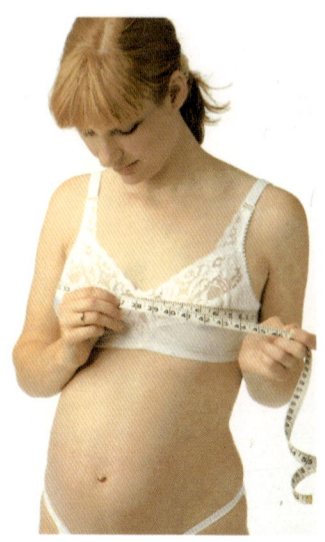

Check your bra size by measuring around your ribcage. For cup size measure around your bust at its fullest.

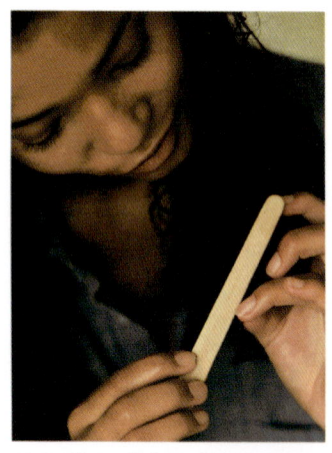

Your nails may be brittle during pregnancy so keep them short to stop them splitting.

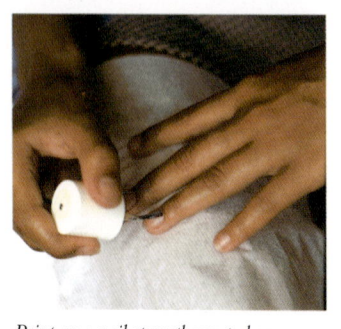

Paint on a nail strengthener to keep your nails strong at this time.

Week 20: Skin Care/Cravings

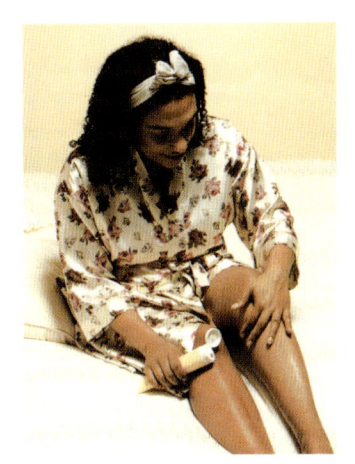

Above: Your legs may ache more with the increased weight you're carrying, so try massaging them with a pleasant body lotion. Right: You can't prevent stretch marks appearing on your stomach, but rubbing in lotion regularly helps to reduce them.

Your growing baby

Vernix, a white greasy substance, is starting to form over the fetus's skin to protect it from the amniotic fluid. This usually wears off before the birth, but sometimes traces of it can be seen. At this stage in your pregnancy the fetus weighs around 340 g/12 oz and measures about 25.5 cm/10 in.

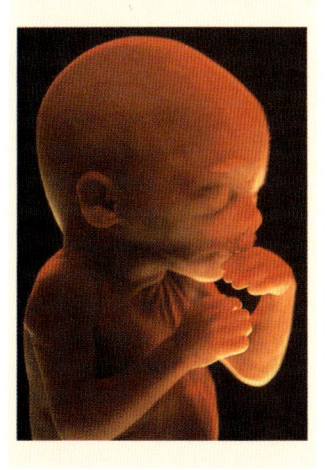

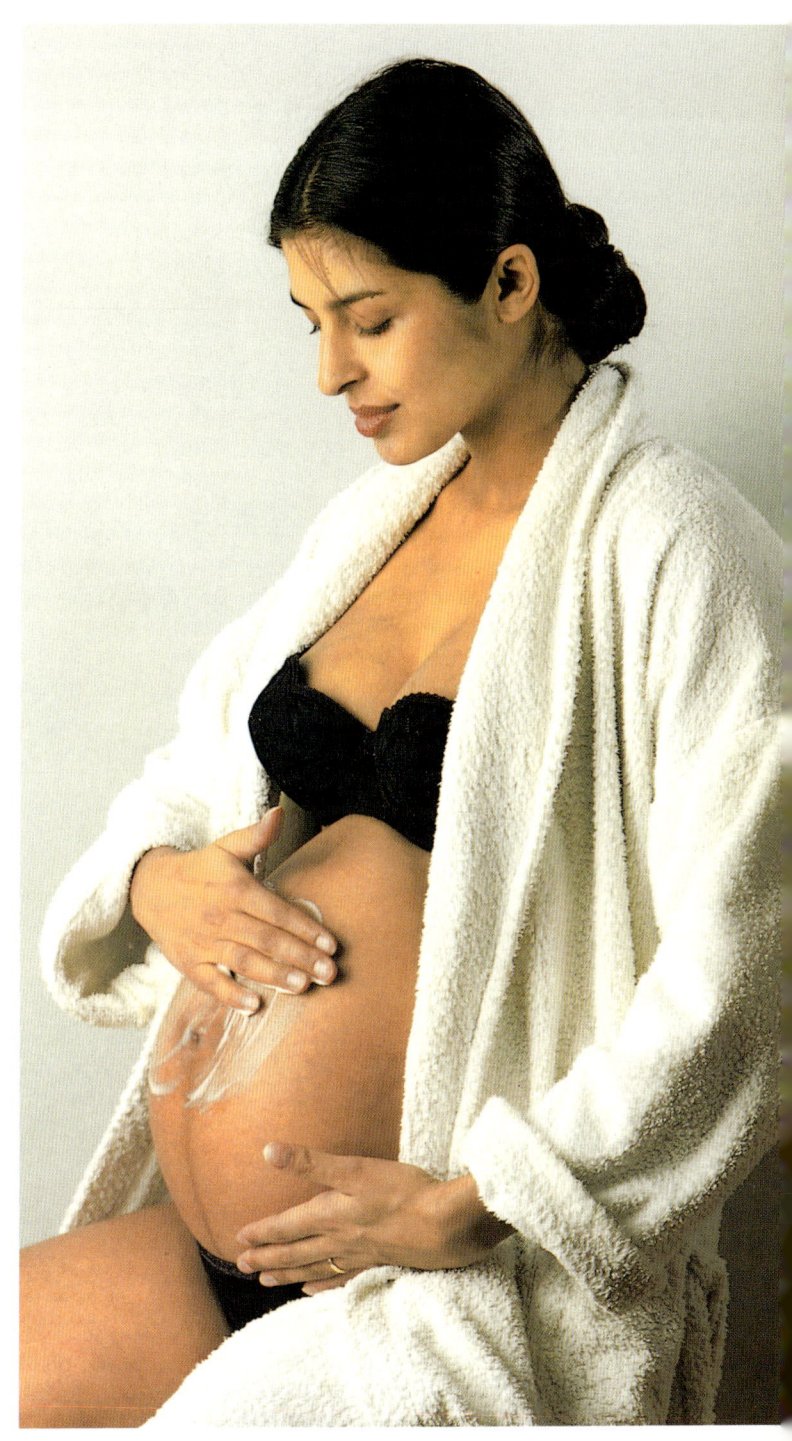

WEEK 21: MINOR COMPLAINTS

You and your body

You should be able to see your abdomen ripple as the fetus moves. You may be feeling slightly breathless as your expanding ribcage pushes upwards, giving your lungs less room. You will probably be feeling energetic so now is the time to tackle things such as planning the nursery.

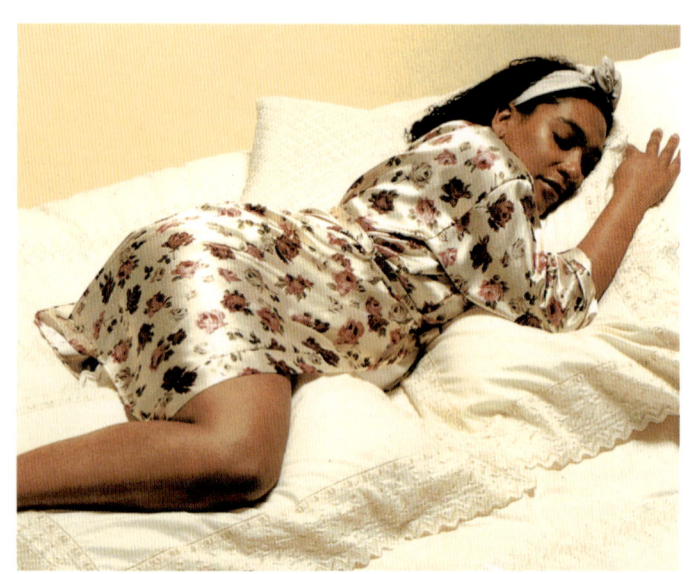

By now you may be experiencing some of the minor problems that occur later in pregnancy. These include:

Heartburn This is a strong burning feeling in your chest which often happens during the last few months of pregnancy. It is usually worse when lying down. Hormones cause the valve at the top of your stomach to relax, which allows stomach acid to pass back into the gullet (oesophagus), causing a burning sensation. Avoid eating spicy and fatty foods. Eating small, but frequent meals will help reduce heartburn. Sleeping propped up at night and drinking a glass of milk before you go to bed will also help ease the discomfort.

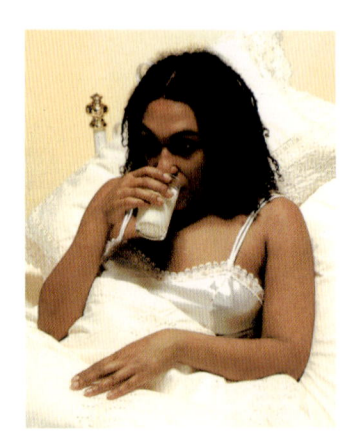

If you are suffering from heartburn, try drinking a glass of milk before you go to sleep at night.

Your doctor may prescribe an antacid if the problem keeps you awake at night. If you buy an over-the-counter remedy always tell the pharmacist that you are pregnant because some of the remedies available are not suitable for use during pregnancy or breast-feeding.

Insomnia Sleeplessness often

Insomnia can be a problem in later pregnancy. If you can't sleep, try supporting your tummy on pillows to make yourself more comfortable.

becomes a problem as your pregnancy progresses because you find it difficult to get comfortable, and you have to make frequent trips to the toilet. Vivid dreams can also be a problem at this time. A bath followed by a warm drink at bedtime will help you relax. It is important to find restful sleeping positions, so use lots of pillows to support your abdomen when you lie on your side. You could also try practising some relaxation techniques.

Itching This often occurs on the areas of skin around the bump and is sometimes accompanied by a rash. Calamine lotion should help relieve the itching and since it is usually caused by sweating, wearing loose clothes made of natural fibres can help prevent it. Severe itching during the last three months of pregnancy could be a warning of pregnancy cholestasis – a rare but potentially dangerous liver disorder – and you should consult your doctor.

Oedema (swelling) This occurs in the feet and ankles and sometimes

Week 21: Minor Complaints

Your growing baby
The fetus is very active now and you will probably be able to feel it kicking quite easily. If this disturbs you at night, stroke your tummy and talk to the fetus because it will be soothed by the sound of your voice. The fetus is now around 28 cm/11 in long and weighs about 390 g/14 oz.

the hands because your body is holding more fluid than normal. By the end of the day this fluid tends to gather in your feet, especially if the weather has been hot or you have been doing a lot of standing. Try to sit or lie with your feet up whenever you can, as this will help reduce the swelling. Wear support tights and comfortable shoes during the day and avoid standing for long periods. You should always tell your midwife or doctor about any swelling that you experience as it could be a sign of pre-eclampsia.

Tiredness The extra weight you carry during late pregnancy can make you feel more tired than usual. It is important to build some regular rest periods into your day when you can sit down with your feet up. If the tiredness you are experiencing feels excessive, you may be suffering from anaemia. Make sure you are getting plenty of iron in your diet by eating lean red meat, whole grains, dark green leafy vegetables, nuts, and pulses. If the feeling still persists then consult your midwife or doctor.

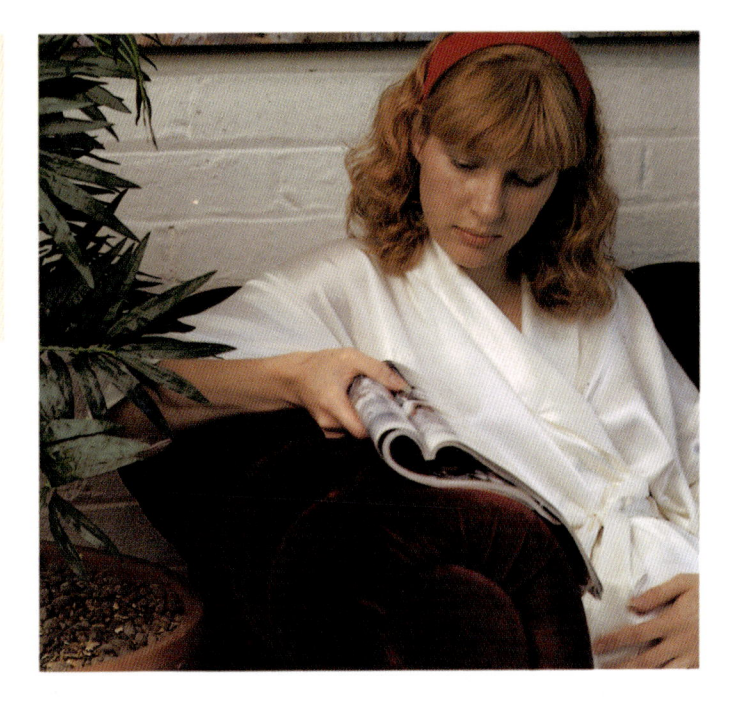

Above: You may well be feeling more energetic than usual at this stage in your pregnancy, but don't forget to give yourself time to sit down and rest.

Below: If your ankles start to swell when you have been on your feet for a while, lie down on the floor with your head supported by a pillow and your feet propped up on several pillows.

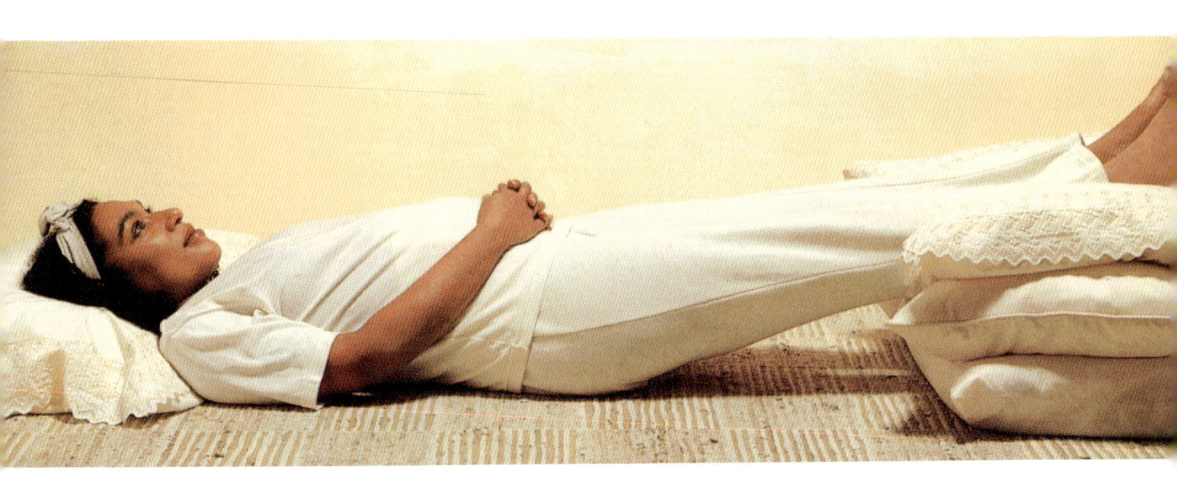

WEEK 22: RELAXATION AND MASSAGE

It is important to be able to relax, both mentally and physically, during pregnancy because this will help you to rest. Knowing how to make your body relax during labour will allow you to work with the contractions rather than against them.

Physical relaxation Start by getting comfortable and make sure that every part of your body is supported. Then concentrate on tensing and relaxing individual parts of your body. Start at your toes and work gradually upwards to your head and then back down to your toes again. By the time you have finished this exercise you should be feeling nice and floppy.

Mental relaxation This requires deep concentration so you need to be completely comfortable and in a quiet place where no one will disturb you. Empty your mind and concentrate on your breathing. Breathe in deeply and hold your breath for a few seconds before letting it out slowly. Once you have established a steady pattern of breathing you should make sure that all your muscles are relaxed, then allow your mind to float away. One way to do this is to imagine that you are floating gently on calm water under a clear blue sky, in tranquil surroundings.

You and your body

Your lower ribs are starting to cause you pain as they get pushed outwards by your growing baby and your expanding uterus. Your ribcage rises by a small amount as it is pushed upward. To minimize the discomfort, try sitting up as straight as you can or lifting your arms above your head. This is an ideal time to investigate the different methods that you can use to ease discomfort now and during labour and birth.

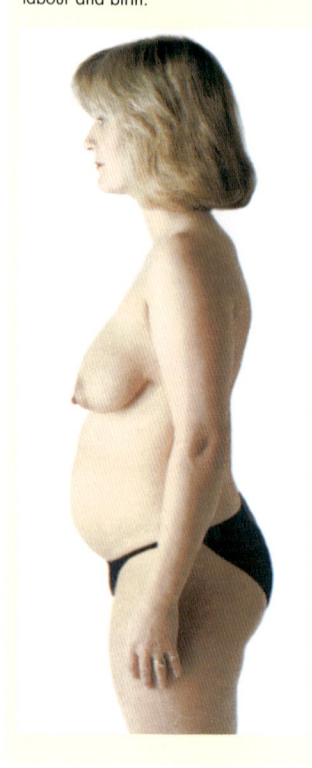

WEEK 22: RELAXATION AND MASSAGE

OTHER TECHNIQUES

Massage is an excellent way of relieving tension. It is best done on bare skin, but if you find your skin is particularly sensitive, it can be carried out through a thin cotton nightdress. Massage strokes should be firm, smooth, and rhythmical.

Aromatherapy massage uses essential oils which are added to a carrier oil before being applied to your skin. Certain essential oils can be dangerous during pregnancy because they may trigger uterine contractions, so you must always get qualified professional advice. Many aromatherapists will not treat a pregnant woman at all. Most of those who will treat expectant mothers will do so only after the sixth month of pregnancy. One effective blend is mandarin oil well diluted (i.e. a maximum solution of one per cent: no more than 10 drops of oil to 50 ml carrier oil) in a sweet almond carrier oil. A well-diluted solution of true lavender, jasmine, and rose in sweet almond oil is also thought to be beneficial during labour and birth.

In acupuncture tiny needles are used to stimulate meridian points situated on the body's energy lines with the aim of rebalancing the energy flow. The treatment can help backache, but some points on the body are thought to stimulate uterine contractions, so it is important to visit a qualified practitioner and let him or her know that you are pregnant.

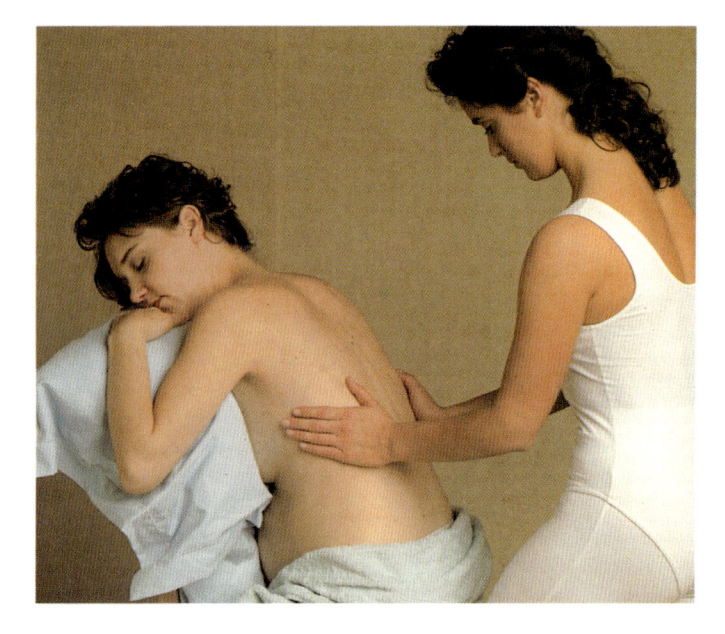

Above: If you are suffering regularly from backache, having a soothing massage from a qualified practitioner can help. With an aromatherapy massage, make sure she chooses oils that will not affect the baby.

Below: Regular massage on your legs will help to relieve any aches and pains that you are experiencing.

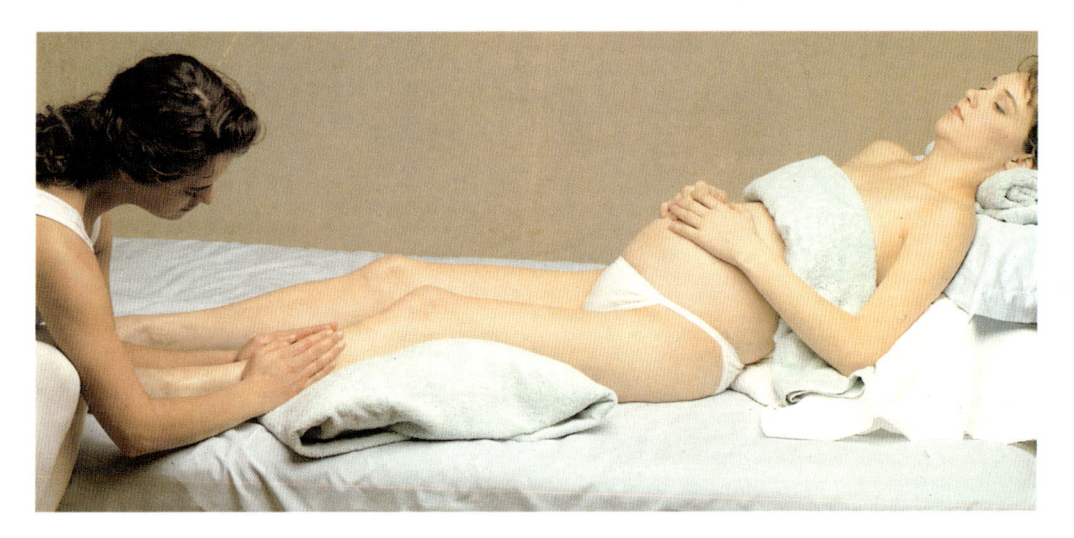

WEEK 23: PREPARING THE NURSERY

You and your body
The baby can be felt through your abdominal wall and the midwife or doctor will palpate your abdomen to see how the baby is lying. You may occasionally feel a pain rather like a stitch down the side of your stomach. This is the uterine muscle stretching and it will go away after you have had a rest.

This is a good time to think of practical things like planning the baby's nursery. Whether you have a spare room which you are going to turn into a nursery, or you intend to make a nursery corner in your own bedroom, you should start getting it ready now while you have the energy.

Before you begin you will need to take into consideration the shape and size of the area so you can work out how much furniture and baby equipment will comfortably fit into it. You should also check whether there are enough electrical sockets; that there is sufficient heating and that the ceiling or wall lights are where you want them. Major changes such as rewiring or putting in another radiator are better done before you start to decorate or carpet the nursery.

Babies enjoy looking at bright, primary colours and big, bold patterns so choose a colourful paint and paper; washable materials will make it easier to keep the walls looking bright and fresh. Transfers, borders, pictures, and mobiles can be used very effectively to brighten up a plain background if you are reluctant to commit yourself to a colour scheme until you know your baby's sex.

Rugs and polished floors look nice but are unsuitable because of the risk of you slipping on them while holding the baby. Any flooring needs to be warm underfoot and non-slip. Sealed cork tiles are ideal because they are warm and any spills can be wiped up without damage to the floor. Fitted carpets and carpet tiles are suitable alternatives, but don't buy expensive carpet because it will probably need replacing after a relatively short time.

An overhead light with a dimmer switch or a specially designed nursery light is very useful for night feeds as it gives out a soft comforting glow which won't startle either of you too much in the middle of the night. A plug or cot light will provide enough illumination for you to check on your sleeping baby, but you will need a brighter light for nappy changing and general care. Avoid any lamps with trailing flexes that you could trip over, and fit all unused electrical sockets with a safety cover.

FINISHING TOUCHES
The room where the baby sleeps must be draught-proof so cover any windows with thick, lined curtains. These will not only keep out any draughts but will also keep the morning light from waking your baby during the summer. Windows need to be fitted with childproof

Planning the nursery for your baby can be enjoyable. You can start to buy some outfits in advance, but remember that you will often be given baby clothes when your baby is born.

Week 23: Preparing the Nursery

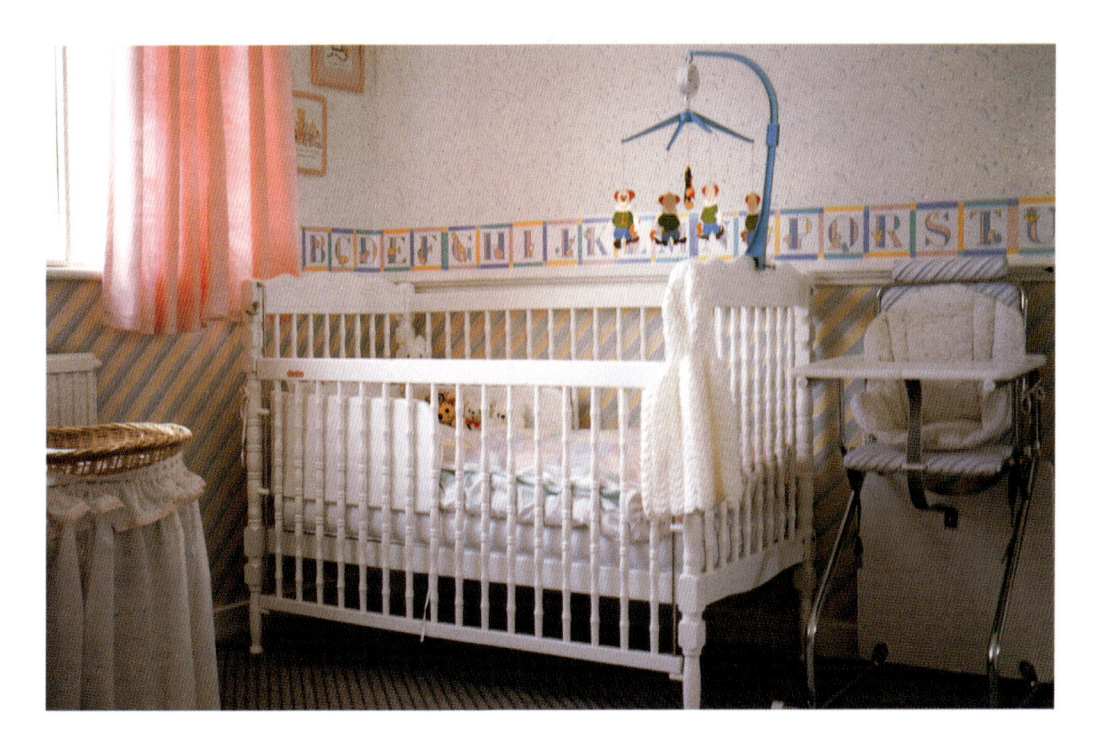

locks and the curtains should be out of reach of the cot. Never place the cot or crib under a window or near radiators. Young babies cannot regulate their own temperature so they need to be kept in a comfortably warm environment at around a constant 18°C/65°F. A special nursery thermometer or a thermostat fitted to the radiator will help ensure that you maintain the room temperature.

Babies actually require very little in the way of furniture. Somewhere to sleep, a cupboard or chest to keep clothes in, and somewhere for changing and storing toiletries and nappies, as well as a chair for you to sit in while you are feeding or rocking the baby, is all that you really need for the first few months. All nursery furniture should be sturdy enough that it can't be pulled over when babies are older and using it for support as they begin to pull themselves up on to their feet.

If you buy secondhand furniture, you will need to make sure that any paint or varnish is non-toxic and lead-free. If you are in any doubt, rub down the furniture well and repaint with safe materials. Also check that there are no broken bits that could harm your baby.

Your growing baby
The fetus is beginning to look as it will at birth, with the head more in proportion to the body. In a boy, the scrotum is now well developed and in a girl the ovaries already contain several million eggs. (These will reduce to around two million at birth and will carry on decreasing until puberty.) The fetus is around 31 cm/12¼ in long and weighs approximately 440 g/ 15½ oz.

When decorating your baby's nursery, bear in mind that babies like bright, primary colours. They also love pretty mobiles.

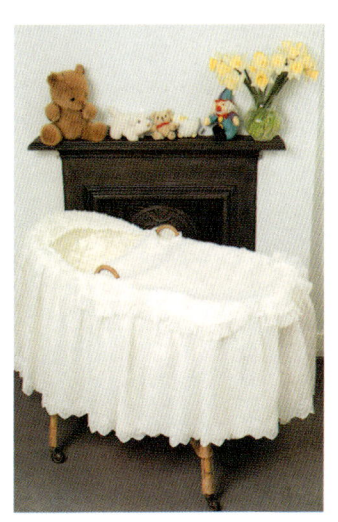

A Moses basket can by kept by or near your bed, and your baby can sleep in it for up to three months.

WEEK 24: BABY CLOTHES AND EQUIPMENT

You and your body
You will noticeably be putting on weight, perhaps as much as 0.5 kg/1 lb per week. Your feet and legs may start to feel the strain of carrying this extra weight, so make sure that you wear comfortable shoes and that you get plenty of rest.

Start planning what you need to buy for your baby so that by the birth you will at least have purchased the major items. If you leave everything until the end of the pregnancy, you may be too tired to enjoy shopping for your baby.

Only buy a few basic first size or newborn garments as your baby will probably rapidly outgrow these. Also, most baby clothes are sized by the approximate age and height of the child and you won't know the size of your child until she is born.

Choose some well-designed baby clothes, which will make your life easier and allow you to dress and undress your baby with the minimum of time and fuss. Clothes with envelope necks or a shoulder fastening will let you slip clothes over the baby's head easily, and poppers up the inside of legs of rompers or all-in-one suits will help to ease the regular nappy changing.

Your new baby will probably get through as many as three changes of clothes a day, so it is a good idea to check the washing instructions on any garment before you buy. These instructions will tell you how best to care for each garment so that you can see whether it is easy-care, or if it will require a lot of attention.

BABY'S TRANSPORT
Before you decide on a pram, buggy, or combination, you need to consider your lifestyle and the various methods of transport you will be

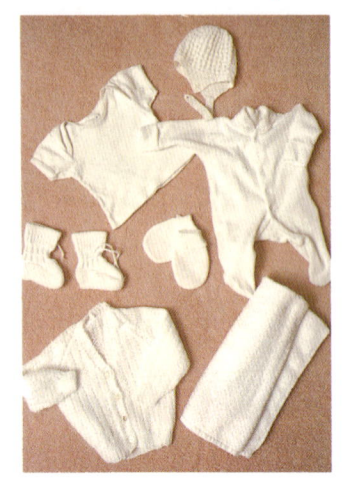

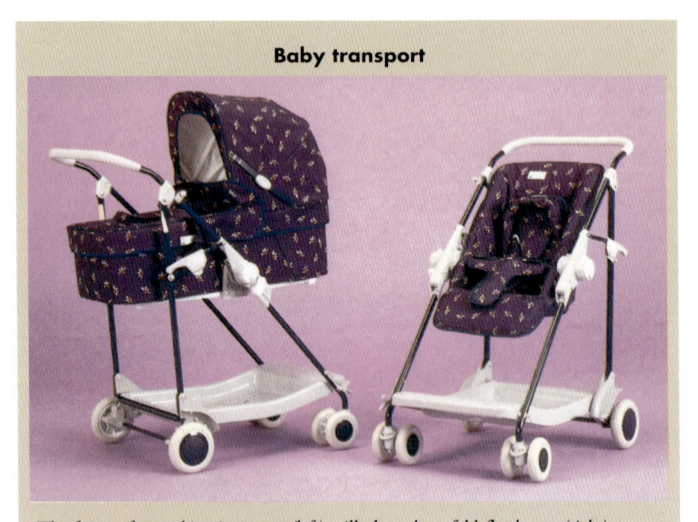

A baby's layette: a bonnet, vest, an all-in-one, mits, bootees, nappy and a cardigan.

Baby transport

The frame of a combination pram (left) will also take a fold-flat buggy (right).

A traditional pram is sturdy with plenty of space for shopping, and it will take a toddler seat. It is probably the best option if you walk everywhere and you are planning to have another child fairly quickly. Generally, prams are unsuitable for cars unless they have a detachable body.

A fold-flat buggy with a reclining seat can be used from babyhood through to toddler stage. Choose one that is light enough to carry on and off public transport.

A 3-in-1 combination converts from pram to push-chair and has a separate baby carrier or carry cot.

Week 24: Baby Clothes and Equipment

using regularly. You also need to think about where it will be stored when not in use. Once you have selected the type most suitable to your needs, ask the shop you order it from to keep it for you until after the baby is born.

If you need a car seat, you can choose between an infant carrier, which is suitable from birth to six months, or a combination seat, which is suitable from birth to around four years. Both types are held securely in place using the existing car seat belts.

Equipment

Whether you buy a cot, Moses basket, or carrycot will probably depend on where your baby is going to sleep and how much space you have. If the baby is going to sleep in your room at first and you haven't much space, think about buying a cot later.

However, when you do purchase a cot make sure that the new mattress you get to go in it is firm. It should also fit snugly into the base of the cot.

You need to have at least six sheets and several lightweight blankets for the cot and another six sheets and at least three more blankets for your chosen pram. You may want to include a cot bumper and throwover as well.

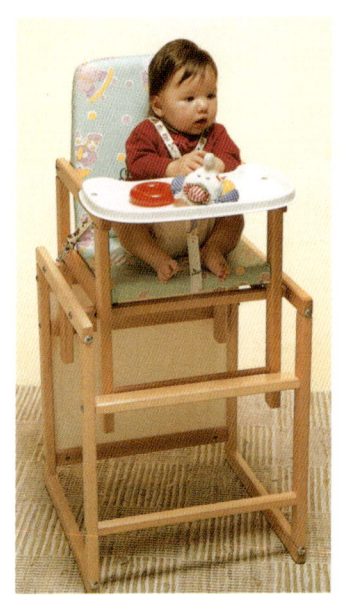

> **Your growing baby**
> Vigorous movements followed by periods of quiet will start to occur as the fetus develops its own waking and resting periods. The pattern that develops now may well continue after the birth so it's a good idea to monitor it for a few days to see how it compares with the sleep pattern once the baby is born. The heartbeat can be heard with an ordinary stethoscope and the fetus can hear you clearly when you speak. It is now around 33 cm/13 in long and weighs about 0.5 kg/1 lb.

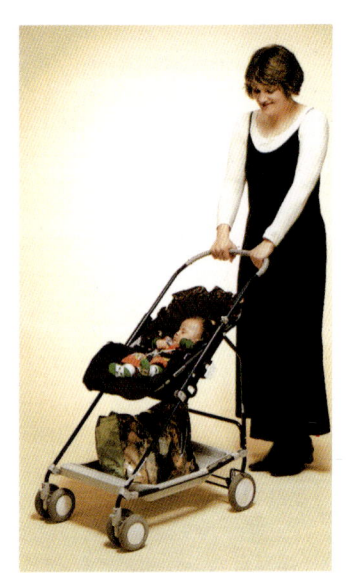

A fold-flat buggy with a parcel shelf can be very useful when you go shopping with your baby.

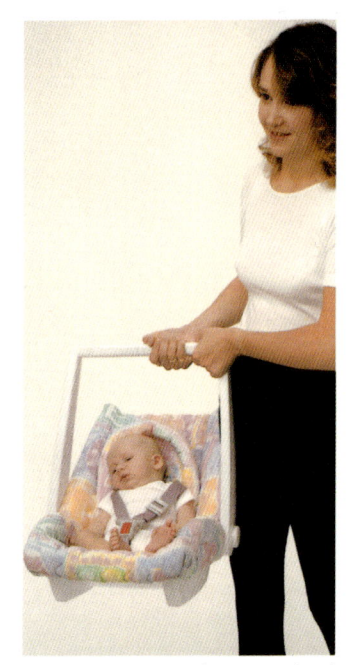

A car seat carrier is easily transported and can be bought in different sizes to suit the age of your baby.

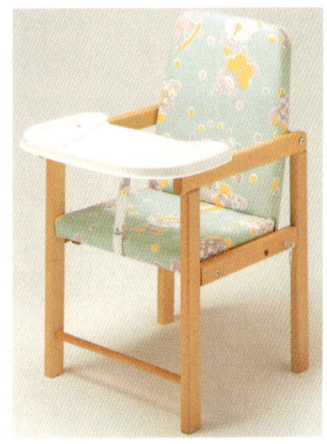

A two-level high chair can be used in the higher position when your baby is young (left) and in the lower position (above) when he is older. Always make sure you fix him in securely.

WEEK 25: FEEDING CHOICES

Now is the time to start thinking about how you are going to feed your baby. Whether to breast- or bottle-feed is a personal and emotional decision and one that you need to feel completely happy about. Before you make up your mind talk it over with your partner and your midwife, and get some first-hand experiences from other mothers.

BREAST-FEEDING
Breast milk is the best possible food for your baby because it contains everything he or she needs in the right proportions, and it changes as the baby grows. It contains antibodies which will help protect the baby and it is easily digestible so less likely to cause stomach upsets. Breast-fed babies are also less likely to develop conditions such as eczema and asthma and are less prone to some infections, such as glue ear.

Breast-feeding has advantages for you as well. Not only is breast milk free and always on "tap", at the correct temperature, it also releases hormones that encourage the uterus to shrink back to its original size more quickly. It uses up calories too, so it will help you get your figure back.

During pregnancy the skin around your nipples will appear darker and raised sebaceous glands will appear as little bumps in the areola, the dark area surrounding the nipple. As your pregnancy progresses the nipples will grow softer. You can help make them more supple by gently massaging them. Take extra care washing and drying your breasts towards the end of pregnancy when they may leak a little, and avoid using soaps that have a drying effect on the skin. You may find that you need to use breast pads to prevent your clothes becoming stained.

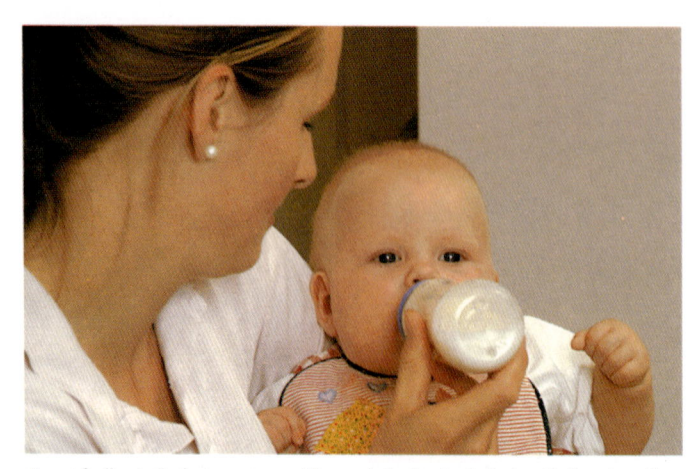

You and your body
You should be looking rosy-cheeked and healthy because of the increase in blood circulation under the skin. Pressure from the growing uterus on the bladder means that you need to make frequent trips to the lavatory. Cramp, heartburn, and backache are often problems now.

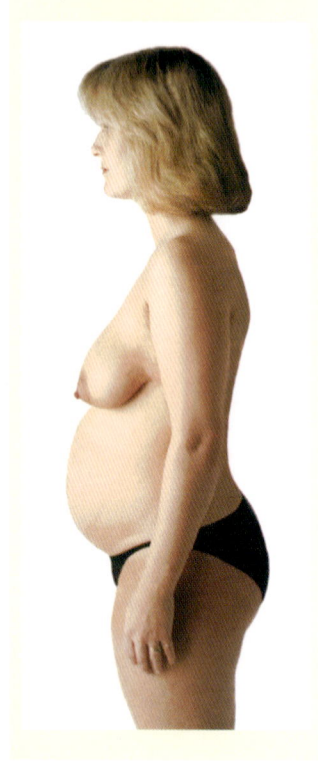

Breast milk is free so the only additional cost involved at first is for nursing bras and breast pads. Choose cotton, front-opening nursing bras, with adjustable straps and fastenings because the size of your breasts will change. Wait until after your 30th week of pregnancy before buying a nursing bra – one that fits you then should fit you after the baby is born.

If you want to be able to express

Breast-feeding is the best way to nourish your baby, but bottle feeds with formula milk can be gradually introduced as he gets older, and can be given by both partners.

WEEK 25: FEEDING CHOICES

milk you will also need a couple of bottles and teats, sterilizing equipment, and possibly a breast pump.

BOTTLE-FEEDING

Formula milk has been specially produced for bottle-fed babies. It contains the right balance of vitamins and minerals that a baby needs to thrive. Formula milk has more protein than breast milk, which means that it takes longer to digest. There are a number of brands to choose from and most are based on cows' milk, although alternatives are available which are designed for children who require special diets for medical reasons. It is very important to follow the instructions when making up formula milk because too much or too little can be harmful. The baby will gradually settle into a routine but until then you will need to respond to his or her hunger just as you would if you were breast-feeding.

One of the main advantages of bottle-feeding is that you and your partner can share the feeds between you, so that you can both use the time when you are feeding to get to know your baby.

Hygiene is very important when you bottle-feed because your baby is not getting protection from the antibodies that he or she would have from breast milk. You will need to take particular care over washing and sterilizing bottles and teats. There are several ways of sterilizing feeding equipment and it is important to choose the method which best suits your needs.

As well as formula milk you will need at least six bottles and teats, with caps, a sterilizing unit or container, a bottle brush, and you may also find a bottle warmer is useful for the night feeds.

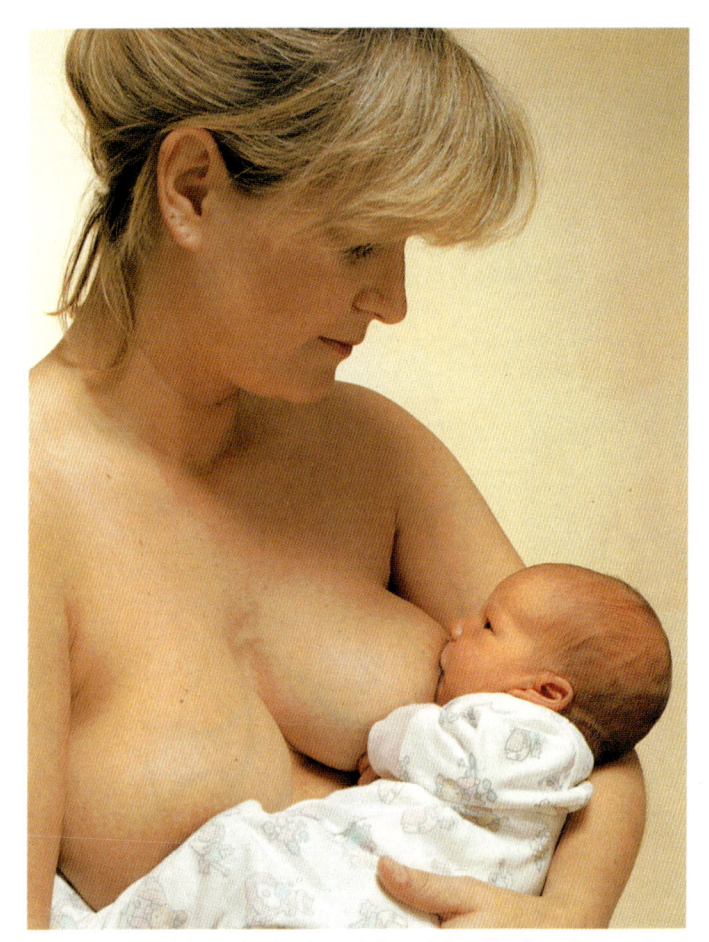

Breast-feeding can help you bond with your baby, and the milk will give her everything she needs, including protection against infection.

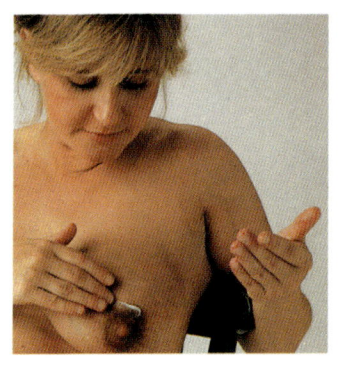

Massaging your nipples in pregnancy will make them more supple for breast-feeding.

Your growing baby

The fetal brain cells continue to develop and become more sophisticated and the bone centres are beginning to harden. The fetus actively practises breathing, inhaling and exhaling amniotic fluid, as more air sacs develop in the lungs. When too much amniotic fluid is swallowed, you may feel a hiccup. The fetus is about 34 cm/13½ in long and weighs around 0.6 kg/1¼ lb.

WEEK 26: PARENTCRAFT CLASSES

You should be about to start parentcraft classes. You may choose one or more of these. Parentcraft classes show you practical techniques such as relaxation, breathing, and postures for labour and birth. The teacher can answer any questions you may have during the last few months of your pregnancy and will be able to give you information on the birth. Your partner will be welcome at some classes and you will find that they are a good way of meeting other pregnant women and sharing mutual anxieties. The hospital and locally run classes are free, but classes such as National Childbirth Trust and Active Birth charge a fee.

HOSPITAL CLASSES

These are run by the hospital where you plan to give birth and usually take place over six to eight weeks, starting around the 28th week. You need to attend the course that is nearest to your expected date of delivery. Some hospitals have a parentcraft teacher, who co-ordinates ante-natal education. You will be taken on a hospital tour so that you can see the labour ward, post-natal ward, and the special care baby unit.

LOCAL CLASSES

These are usually run by a midwife or a health visitor attached to your doctor's surgery or health centre and take place over six to eight weeks.

You and your body

If you are working you need to decide when you are going to stop. Remember that you should notify your employer in writing three weeks before you intend to leave. If you think you may qualify for maternity allowance from the DSS, now is the time to apply for it. If you haven't started taking regular exercise you should now, because this will help prepare your body for the rigours of labour.

Active birth classes

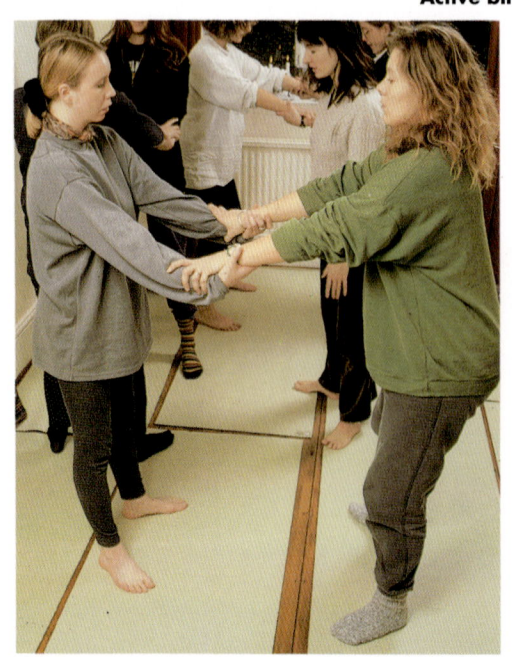

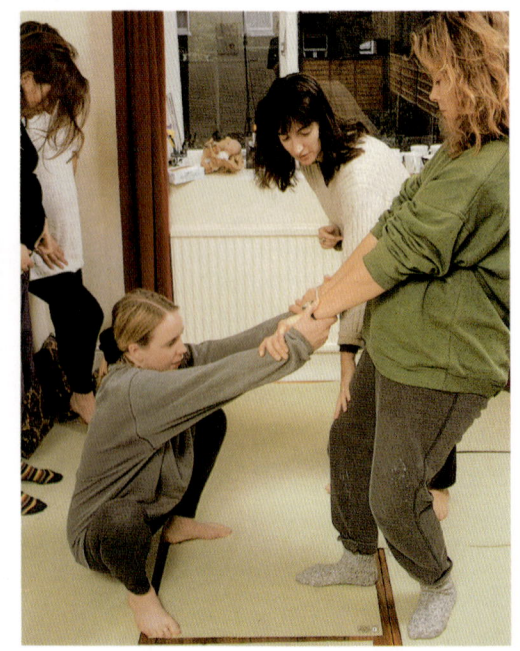

NATIONAL CHILDBIRTH TRUST (NCT)

NCT classes are privately run, usually by mothers who have been trained by the NCT. They need to be booked early because they are deliberately kept small and they become fully booked very quickly. Although everything covered on the hospital and local parentcraft courses is included on the NCT course, the classes are more discussion-based and there are no rigid relaxation and breathing techniques. You are taught a variety of skills for dealing with labour and the birth, from which you can choose when the time comes.

ACTIVE BIRTH CLASSES

These are privately run weekly classes that concentrate on the physical preparation for labour and birth. You are taught a range of yoga-based stretching exercises as well as breathing and relaxation techniques. These classes are mainly for women, with a special session for fathers, and you can join them at any time during your pregnancy.

BREATHING TECHNIQUES

Controlled breathing is important during labour and you need to practise the breathing exercises you will be taught at your classes. Breathing needs to be slow and smooth with deep breaths, inhaled through your nose and exhaled through your mouth. A long slow breath at the beginning of each contraction will help oxygenate your blood and this may help relieve any pain caused by lack of oxygen to the muscles of your uterus. Oxygen is also carried in the blood flowing through the placenta into the umbilical cord, so if you do not get enough, your baby will suffer a shortage too.

During contractions you will be concentrating on each outward breath as this will help you to relax your muscles. It will be important not to over-breathe during the second stage of labour, because this may make you feel dizzy and light-headed. If you do find yourself needing to breathe more quickly then you should concentrate on making each breath as light as possible.

Your growing baby

Although still appearing rather scrawny, the fetus is beginning to lay down fat under the skin. This fat will help regulate body temperature now and after the birth. The fetus is around 35 cm/13¾ in long and weighs approximately 0.7 kg/1½ lb.

Gentle yoga-based exercises are ideal preparation for labour and help you to get ready physically and emotionally, so that you are in tune with the demands on your body. They should always be done under qualified supervision. Exercises include going down into a squatting position (far left and left) in anticipation of labour; massage, which particularly helps if you've got sciatica (below left), and stretching to ease pressure at the base of the spine (below right).

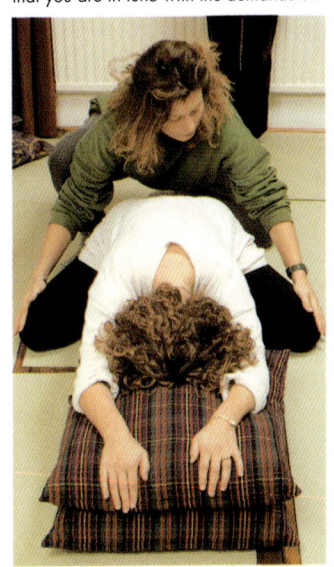

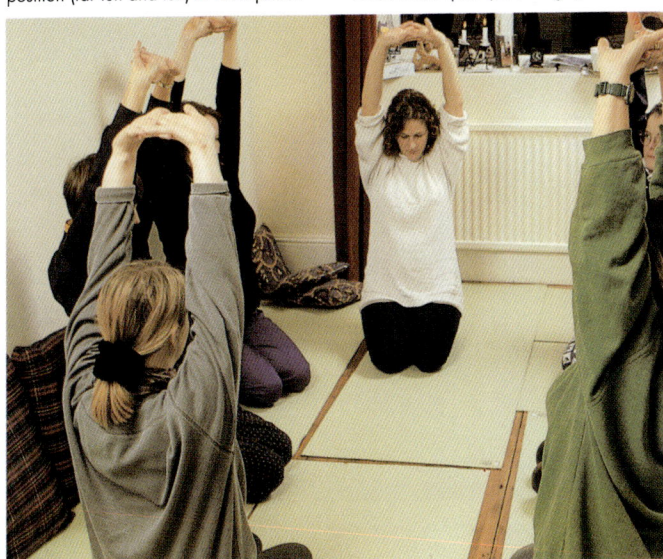

THE THIRD TRIMESTER

WEEK 27: CHOICES IN CHILDBIRTH

Now that you have entered the third trimester you should start planning the kind of birth that you want. If you are having a hospital birth, you will need to discover what facilities are on offer and then try to plan the birth around them. Although nowadays hospitals do try to accommodate a mother's wishes, not all are able to offer every type of birth. If you want an active or water birth, you will have to find out whether it is possible at your hospital. If you are having a home birth then having an active birth or a water birth in a hired pool is easier to arrange. However, you need to remember that if complications occur during labour any decisions you make now may have to be changed.

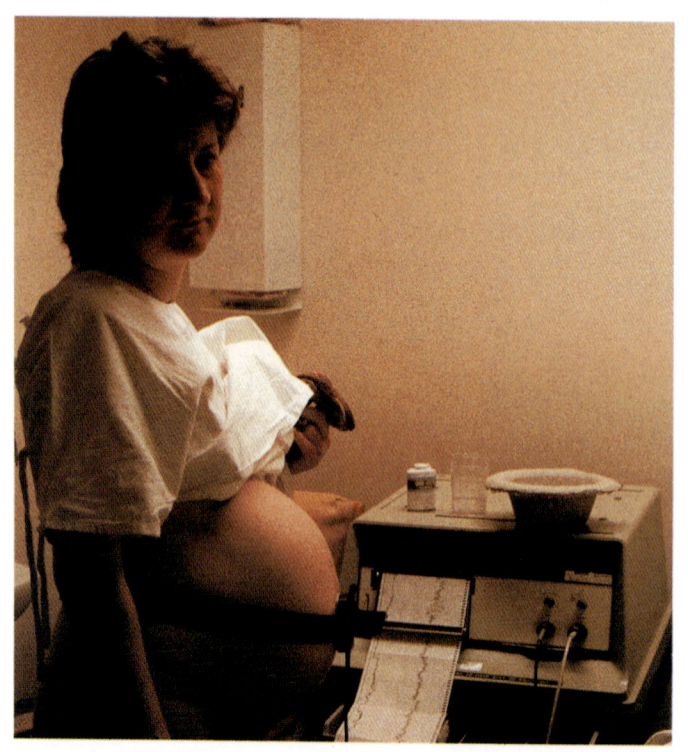

When you give birth in hospital, special straps might well be put round your bump to attach you to a monitor that checks the strength of your baby's heartbeat.

You and your body

You will be getting noticeably larger and will have put on weight around your chest as well as your breasts. Make sure that you are wearing the correct size of maternity bra. Avoid lying on your back too much because this may make you feel faint, as the enlarged uterus presses directly against blood vessels.

NATURAL BIRTH
This is when you go through labour and birth without any of the medical procedures that often alter the natural rhythm of labour. Natural childbirth involves the use of breathing and relaxation techniques and sometimes homeopathic remedies.

WATER BIRTH
You spend part of your time in a birth pool, which is filled with warm water, and give birth either outside the pool or in the water. The warm water eases contractions, making them less painful, and helps you to relax. Although there is no evidence to prove that there is an increased risk of complications if you actually have your baby in the water, you should still talk to your midwife or doctor before planning to do this.

ACTIVE BIRTH
This means that you are free to move and walk about during labour. Keeping mobile allows the contractions to be more effective. Being in an upright position helps the baby's circulation and encourages the baby to rotate into the best position for

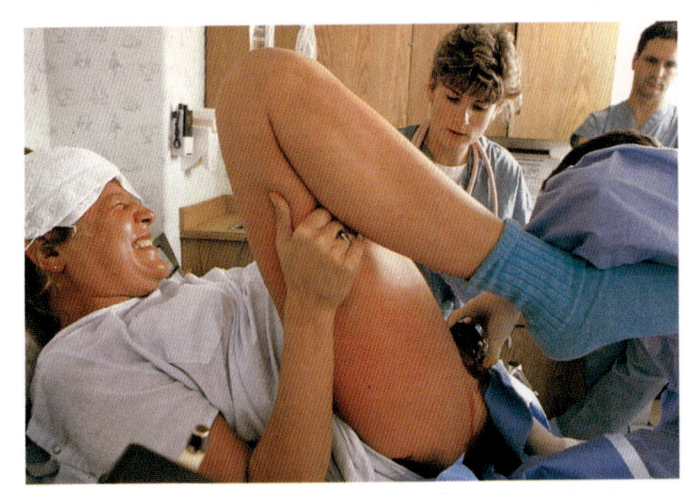

WEEK 27: CHOICES IN CHILDBIRTH

In a natural birth you go through labour without painkillers, using only relaxation methods and maybe homeopathic treatments.

delivery. Gravity aids the baby's descent, and giving birth in a squatting or kneeling position increases the size of the pelvic outlet.

HIGH-TECH BIRTH
Labour is controlled by medical methods such as induction, where labour is started artificially using chemical substances, or the waters are broken manually. Painkilling drugs are used and an episiotomy (a surgical incision in the perineum to allow passage of the fetal head when there is some fear that the perineum will otherwise be torn) may be done to enlarge the birth canal.

CAESAREAN BIRTH
This is when the baby is delivered through an incision that is made through the wall of the abdomen into the uterus. It is done under a general anaesthetic, or sometimes with an epidural (an injection that deadens pain only in the lower spine). If an epidural is used you will be awake during the delivery, although a screen is placed across your body so that you don't actually see what is happening. You will be given your baby to hold as soon as it is born. After the birth, the incisions are stitched and you will be kept in hospital for about five days. A Caesarean may be chosen if the reasons that make it necessary are evident before labour begins. This is known as an elective Caesarean. If it is decided on after labour has started, it is known as an emergency Caesarean. Reasons for a Caesarean include abnormal presentation of the baby (that is, not head-first towards the cervix), fetal distress where the baby suffers from lack of oxygen, and high blood pressure in the mother.

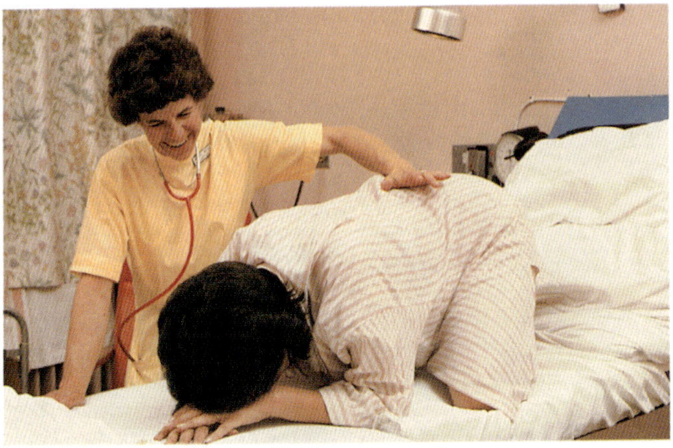

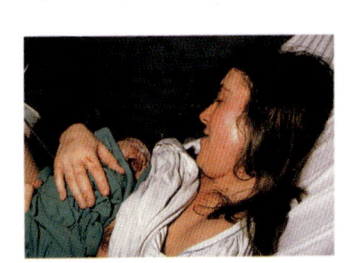

When you hold your newborn baby in your arms all the hard work of labour will seem worthwhile.

An active birth involves moving around in labour and adapting different positions that will help your baby's descent.

Your growing baby
The fetus's eyes are open and it will be able to see light through the skin of your abdomen. It will have started to practise sucking and may even be able to suck its thumb or fist. The fetus is now about 36 cm/14¼ in long and weighs about 0.8 kg/1¾ lb.

WEEK 28: THE BIRTHPLAN

Some hospitals include a special form with your notes, on which you can make a written plan of the way you would like your labour and birth to be managed. If you haven't received one of these, talk to your midwife about drawing up your own plan. Even if there are still things concerning labour or the birth about which you are undecided, writing out a plan will help you focus on the type of birth you want. It will also give you the opportunity to discuss the birth in detail with your partner.

When drawing up your birthplan it is important to remember that there is no right or wrong way to give birth. Your plan should reflect what you feel is right for you, while taking into account your medical history as well as the facilities available at the place where you are going to have your baby.

A birthplan is a guide to how you would like things to be, but in the event of a problem this ideal may become totally impractical so you will need to be flexible. Once you have finalized your birthplan ask for a copy to be kept with your notes so that the doctor and midwife who attend you during labour have it to hand. Keep a copy for yourself so that your birth partner can refer to it if necessary.

BIRTH PARTNER
Although your partner will be encouraged to be with you during labour, you may prefer to have another woman as your actual birth partner, especially if your partner is

You and your body
Your breasts are producing colostrum, the fluid which precedes breast milk. If your breasts are leaking put breast pads or folded tissues inside your bra. If you have an ante-natal appointment you will probably have a second blood test to check for anaemia. If you are anaemic, iron supplements may be offered.

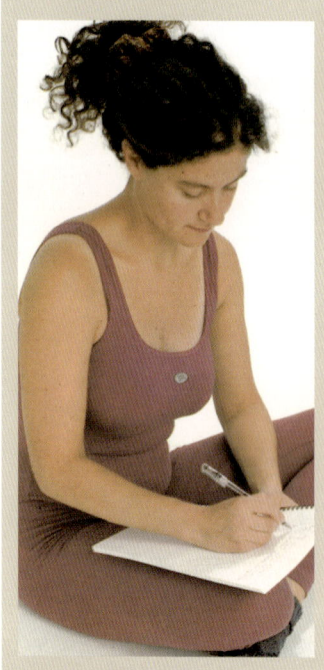

Write a birthplan with your choices.

Birthplan checklist
The following questions will help you prepare your own birthplan.
- Whom do you wish to have with you during labour – your partner, your mother, a friend? You can choose more than one birth partner.
- Can your birth partner remain with you if you have to have a Caesarean or forceps delivery?
- Are there special facilities such as a birthing pool or bean bags available to you?
- Do you want to be free to move around during labour, or would you rather be constantly monitored while staying in bed?
- Is there any special position you want to use for the birth?
- Do you wish to wear your own clothes during labour and the birth?
- Would you like music, soft lighting, massage or other therapies to help you cope with getting through labour?
- How do you feel about pain relief? If you want to manage without any, you will need to make sure that everyone knows. If you want pain relief which sort do you want?
- Are you prepared to have an episiotomy if it is required, or would you rather tear naturally?
- Do you want your baby placed straight onto your abdomen or do you want him or her cleaned up first?
- Are you going to breast-feed? If so, do you want to put your baby to the breast immediately?
- Do you want an injection to help deliver the placenta or would you prefer to wait for it to be delivered naturally after the birth?
- How soon after the birth would you like to go home, assuming that there are no complications?

WEEK 28: THE BIRTHPLAN

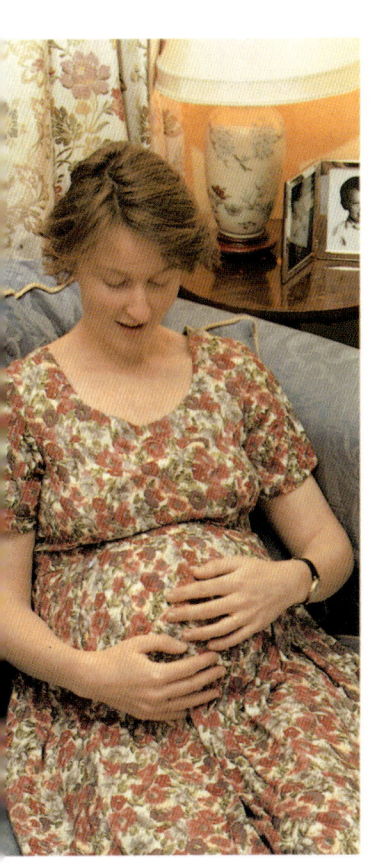

Once you've made your birthplan and put your feelings on your baby's birth in writing, you will feel happier.

worried that he may not be able to cope with seeing you in pain. Whatever you decide, make sure you talk about it together so that there are no misunderstandings and you don't get upset about the final choice.

Your growing baby

Now fully formed, the fetus would be viable if it were born at 28 weeks, although the body systems are still very immature. The heart is beating at a rate of around 150 beats a minute. The fetus weighs around 0.9 kg/2 lb.

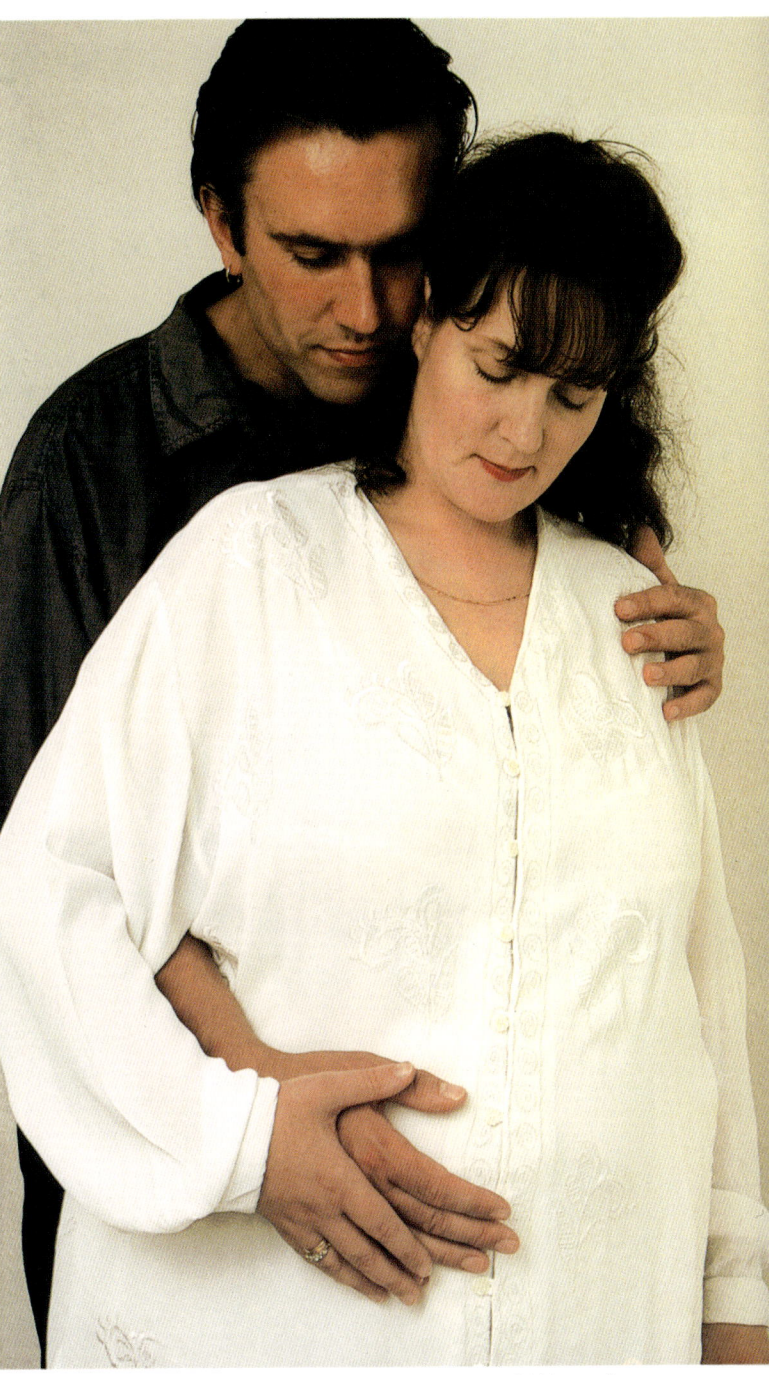

If your partner is worried about being with you during a long or painful labour, talk it through with him and make your feelings known if you're counting on his support.

WEEK 29: SPECIAL CARE

If you suffer from a medical condition or blood disorder your pregnancy will require careful managing. Your doctor will need to monitor your progress and you may have to have special ante-natal checks. If there is a possible problem, you will be offered another scan during the last trimester, which will clearly show the fetus's breathing movements, how it is lying, and the position of the placenta.

Anaemia is caused by an abnormally low level of red corpuscles in the blood and is treated with iron supplements. You can build up your body's store of iron by eating a diet which includes red meat, whole grains, dark green leafy vegetables, nuts, and pulses. Liver is not recommended because of the high levels of vitamin A, which could be toxic. A second blood test is done in late pregnancy to check for anaemia.

Kidney infection is usually caused by bacterial infection and you should contact your doctor if you think you have a kidney infection. Symptoms are pain, frequent urination accompanied by a burning sensation, and occasionally blood in the urine. Other symptoms you may experience include back pain, high fever, chills, nausea, and vomiting.

You and your body
You will probably be able to feel the fetus's bottom and feet as it moves around. The fetus will be putting pressure on your stomach and diaphragm now and you will need to sit down and rest more often.

Placenta praevia is a rare condition which usually occurs when a woman has had more than one child. The placenta is situated low in the uterus so that it blocks, or partially blocks, the cervix. The pressure of the fetus on the placenta may cause painless bleeding any time after 28 weeks. If this happens, you may have to stay in hospital until after your baby is born. If the obstruction is particularly severe, your baby may need to be delivered by Caesarean.

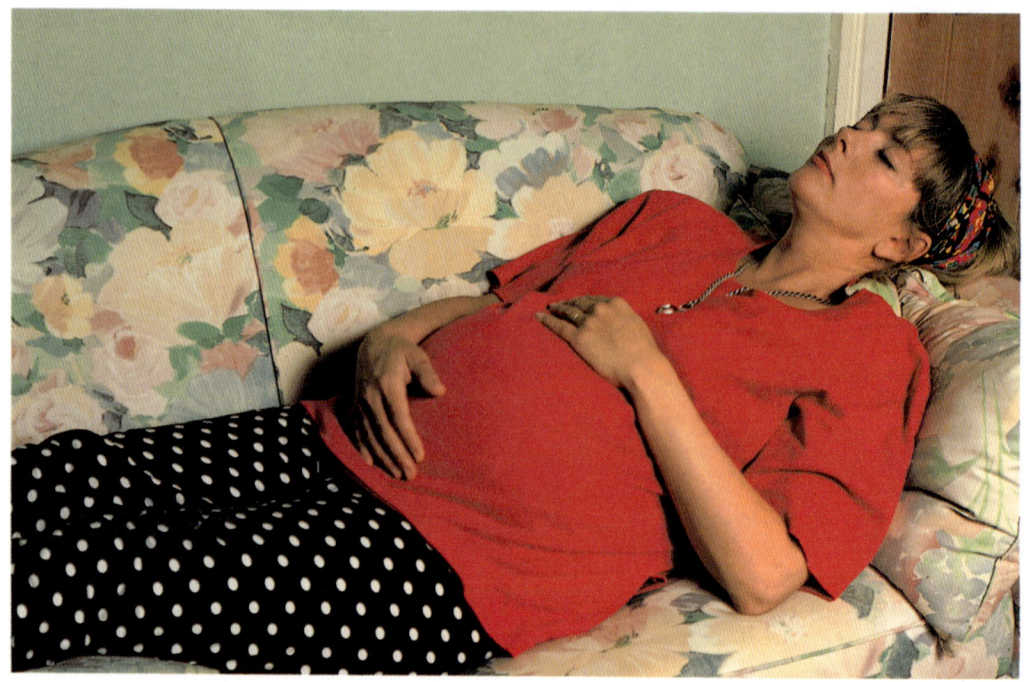

As your baby starts to put pressure on your stomach, you'll need to lie down more often to rest.

Week 29: Special Care

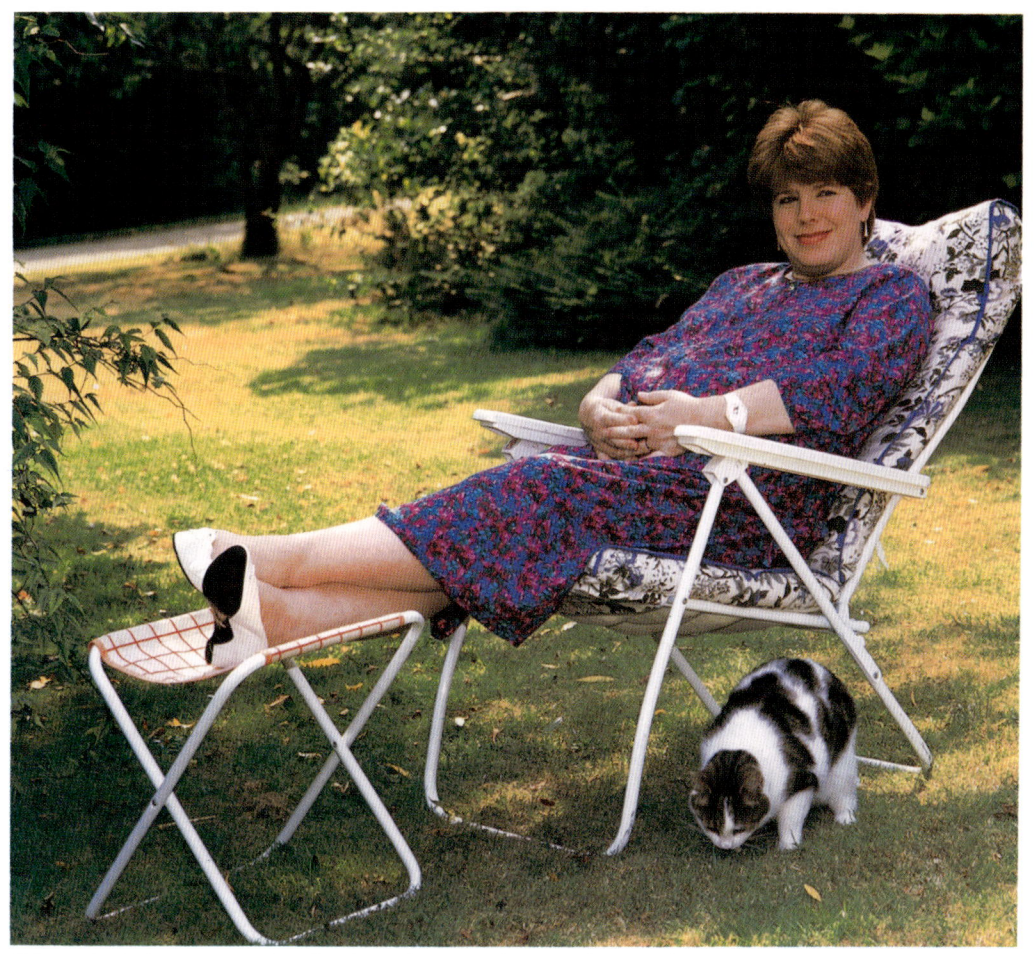

If the weather is pleasant, you might well prefer to take your regular rests in the garden, but remember to support your legs.

Abruptio placentae is when part of the placenta comes away from the wall of the uterus causing some abdominal pain and bleeding. You should call the doctor immediately. The fetus could be at risk if a large part of the placenta has come away, because it will be deprived of necessary oxygen and nutrients. Sometimes a blood transfusion is necessary and in late pregnancy the baby may be delivered by Caesarean. If only a small part of the placenta has come away, you will need to have complete bedrest until the bleeding stops.

Placental insufficiency occurs when the placenta doesn't function efficiently and the fetus grows more slowly than normal because of lack of nourishment. If this happens, you will be told to rest so that the blood flow from the placenta to the fetus can improve. A urine test will also be taken to see whether the health of the fetus is being affected and whether induction is going to be necessary for the birth.

Your growing baby

The fetus is filling almost all the space in your uterus and its head is now more or less in proportion with the rest of the body. The eyebrows and eyelashes are fully grown and the fetus has quite a lot of hair which is still growing. The eyes, which can now open and close, are beginning to focus. The fetus weighs around 1 kg/2¼ lb and is about 38 cm/ 15 in long.

WEEK 30: TRAVEL/BACKACHE

There is no reason why you shouldn't travel during pregnancy, but during the later stages you should check with your doctor if you are going abroad. Airlines may not be willing to take you once you are past 28 weeks because of the risk of a premature labour occurring.

If you want to fly you will need to check with the airline before you book a ticket; the airline may insist on a medical certificate stating that it is safe for you to travel. If you wish to visit a country where immunization is required, you will have to get medical advice because some vaccines should be avoided completely in pregnancy.

You will probably want to avoid long car journeys towards the end of pregnancy because you may find them uncomfortable. When travelling by car it is important to wear your seat belt so that it fits neatly across your thighs and above your abdomen, but not across the middle. If the belt was worn across your body it could possibly cause damage to your baby if you were involved in a car accident.

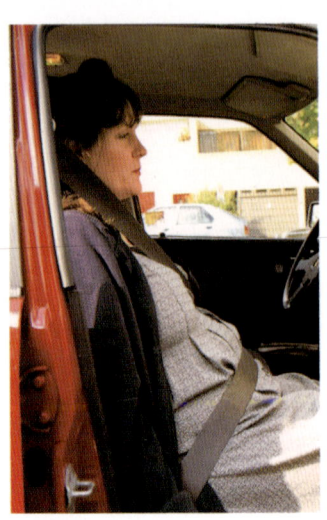

Backache

This can be particularly troublesome during the last months of pregnancy. Hormones have softened your ligaments and the additional weight you are carrying inevitably puts a strain on your stomach muscles, which in turn puts strain on your back muscles. If the backache you are suffering is particularly severe, always check it out with your doctor because it can indicate the presence of a kidney infection.

You and your body

You will feel larger and clumsier now and your movements will be slower. It is important to try to maintain good posture to prevent backache. You may have problems sleeping and become a bit breathless if you walk too fast or climb stairs.

Ease upper backache by lying flat on a firm surface with pillows under your head and knees. Lower backache can be helped by kneeling on all fours, with your back straight and your hands and knees well apart, then dropping your head and arching your back. Repeat this exercise several times.

You can help to avoid backache by wearing low-heeled shoes and trying not to hollow your back when you are standing. When you sit down, put a cushion in the small of your back; when you get out of a chair, push yourself right to the edge before attempting to stand up.

A firm mattress will help when you are lying down; when you get up from the lying position, roll over onto your side and then push yourself slowly up. If you have to bend down, always bend your body from the knees and then squat down to pick up anything from the floor.

Your growing baby

The fetus is beginning to move about less vigorously now because it has less space to move around in the uterus. To get comfortable it is likely to adopt a curled-up position with arms and legs crossed. The fetus is now about 39 cm/15½ in long and weighs around 1.1 kg/2½ lb.

Don't fasten your seat belt over your bump as your baby could be damaged in a accident.

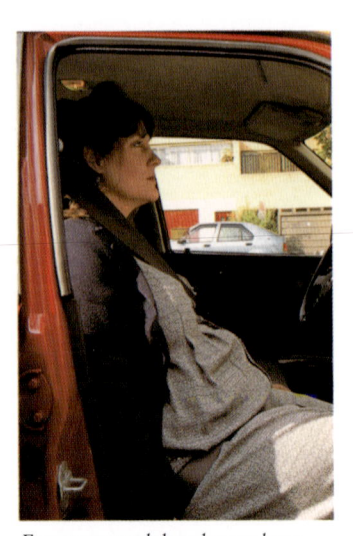

Fasten your seat belt under your bump and across your thighs to protect your baby.

Week 30: Travel/Backache

Bending in pregnancy

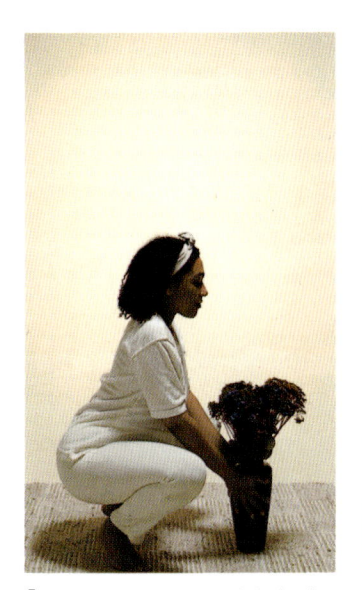

1 In later pregnancy particularly, bend your knees, not from the waist, and pick up the object when you are squatting.

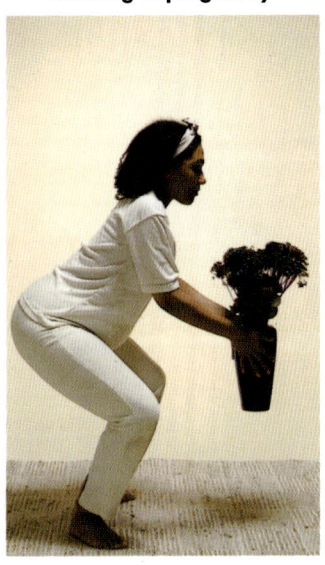

2 As you get up from the squatting position, keep your back straight and lift up the object at arm's length.

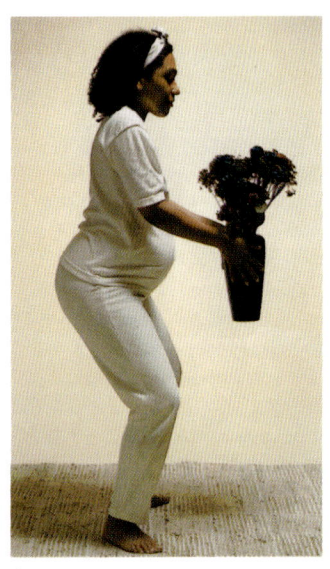

3 As you gradually become upright, straighten your bent knees without making any jerky movements.

How to relieve backache

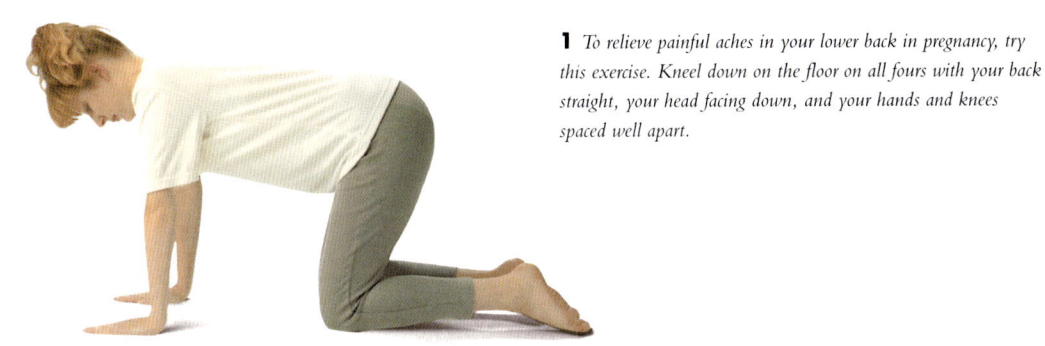

1 To relieve painful aches in your lower back in pregnancy, try this exercise. Kneel down on the floor on all fours with your back straight, your head facing down, and your hands and knees spaced well apart.

2 Drop your head right down and arch your back to stretch out the painful muscles, hold for several seconds, then release, raising your head up again. Repeat the exercise several times for the best relief.

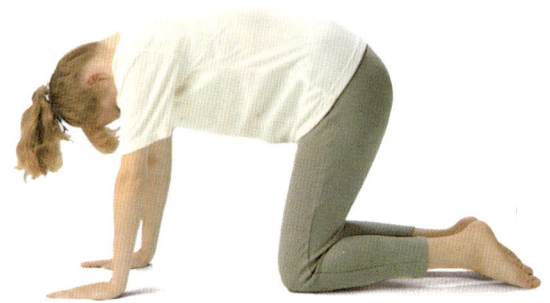

WEEK 31: DEALING WITH DISCOMFORT

You and your body
Breathlessness may be more of a problem now, especially if you overdo things. Try to get as much rest as possible and slow down any exercise regime to a pace that suits you. If your breasts feel uncomfortable when you go to bed, wear a maternity or specially designed sleep bra at night.

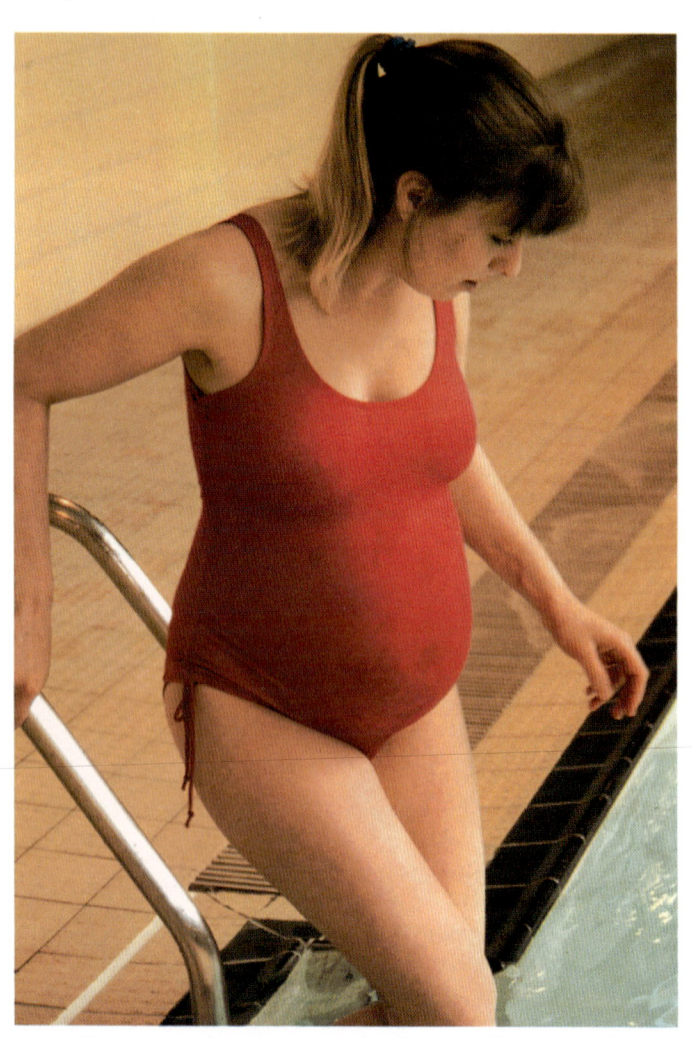

The fetus is getting quite big and will be putting pressure on your diaphragm, which may mean that you are now finding it more difficult to breathe. This breathlessness should pass once the fetus's head drops into the pelvis and becomes engaged in a few weeks' time. Try sitting and standing as straight as possible, and put some extra pillows behind your shoulders when you are in bed.

You are likely to need a larger size of bra towards the end of pregnancy and the one that you buy now should fit you after the baby is born. If you are intending to breast-feed, buy a front-opening nursing bra that will be suitable both now and after the birth.

Choose a bra with wide adjustable straps and fastenings and which has a broad supportive band under the cups. Make sure that the cups fit comfortably and do not gape under the arms. Buy one made from cotton or a cotton mixture that will be more comfortable to wear, and allow your skin to breathe properly, particularly in hot weather.

BRAXTON HICKS CONTRACTIONS
During pregnancy you will experience contractions which may be uncomfortable but are not usually painful. These are known as Braxton Hicks contractions, which tighten the muscles of the uterus about every 20 minutes throughout pregnancy, although you have probably not been aware of them during the early months. In the last weeks of pregnancy these contractions become more noticeable as they begin to prepare the uterus for labour by drawing up the cervix and making it thinner. When you have

Exercise like swimming, where you are supported in the water, will keep you fit in late pregnancy. It will also relieve backache as the swimming motion will stretch the back muscles.

Week 31: Dealing With Discomfort

these contractions, practise your breathing techniques for labour.

Kick counts

You can check on your baby's well-being by keeping a count of the fetal movements. If there is any concern about the fetus's development you may be asked to keep a kick chart recording the first 10 movements each day. For your own peace of mind you should be aware of these movements so that if for any reason they become less frequent, or even stop altogether, you will notice immediately. If you are ever concerned about lack of movement, seek some medical advice immediately because it could indicate some trouble with the fetus.

As your pregnancy progresses and the fetus gets bigger it has less room to manoeuvre, so movements will be more noticeable, but less frequent. By the end of your pregnancy the fetus will probably move between 10 and 12 times in a 12-hour period.

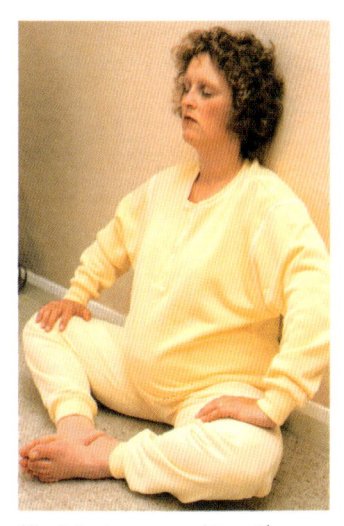

Try sitting in a yoga position with your back straight to alleviate the pressure your baby is putting on your diaphragm.

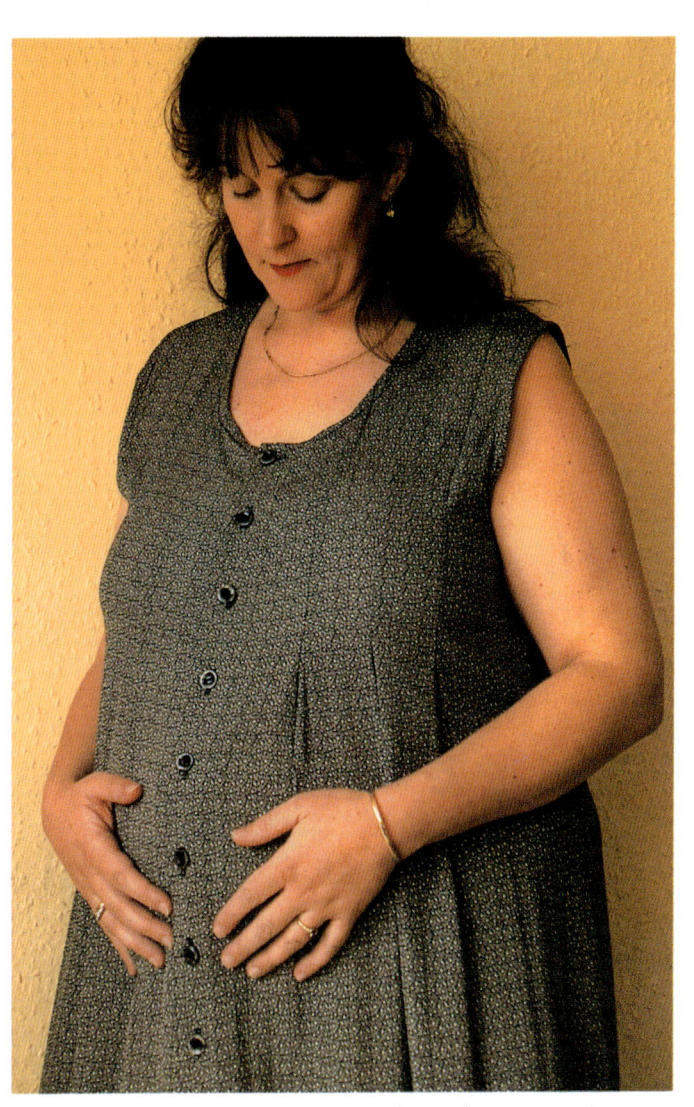

Keep a kick count of your baby's movements on a chart, so that you can monitor any noticeable changes and seek medical help if you feel it is necessary.

Your growing baby

The organs are almost completely developed, apart from the lungs which are still not fully mature. The brain is still growing and the nerve cells and connections are now working. A protective sheath is developing around the nerve fibres so that messages travel faster, enabling the fetus to learn more. It can feel pain, will move if prodded and you can feel it jump at loud noises. The fetus is around 40 cm/15¾ in long and weighs about 1.4 kg/3 lb.

WEEK 32: POSITIONS FOR LABOUR

It is a good idea to practise some of the positions that will help you through the different stages of labour. During the first stage you should try to stay upright and keep active. Being upright will make your contractions stronger and more efficient. It will also allow gravity to keep the baby's head pressed down, which will help your cervix to dilate faster so that labour is speeded up. Remaining active will give you more control over labour so that you should feel less pain. If you are lying down, your uterus presses on the large blood vessels running down your back and this can reduce the blood flow through the placenta to and from the baby. If you feel you want to lie down during labour, try to position yourself on your side rather than on your back.

COPING WITH CONTRACTIONS
You should aim to give the fetus as much room as possible in your pelvis and the best way to achieve this is by keeping your knees well apart and leaning forward so that the uterus tilts away from your spine. During the first-stage contractions it may help to lean against your partner, or if you prefer you can kneel down resting your arms and head on a cushion on the seat of a chair. If you find being upright tiring, try kneeling on all fours. This allows you to keep the weight of the fetus off your lower back. By the time your contractions are coming every few minutes you may want to adopt a squatting position, or you could try kneeling forward onto a pile of cushions or a bean bag with your legs wide apart. It may help if your partner massages your back while you are in this position.

When you reach the second stage you'll want to find a comfortable position for the birth. If you lie on your back you will literally have to push the baby uphill. If you remain upright your abdominal muscles will work more efficiently as you bear down, and gravity will help the baby out. Try squatting, supported on both sides, or with your partner supporting you from behind, so that your pelvis is at its widest and you have control over the pelvic floor

You and your body
If you work, you may have left by now or will have a date when you are going to leave. Enjoy the last weeks of your pregnancy and spend time singing and talking to your baby. You may find the fetal movements uncomfortable now that it is so much bigger. Occasionally, you may feel its feet getting stuck under your ribs.

Labour positions

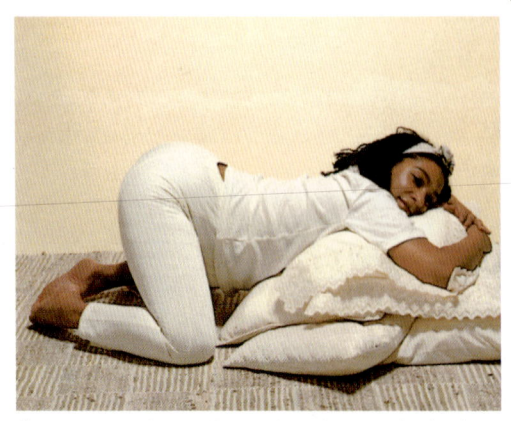

1 *Relax on all fours by flopping forward onto a pile of cushions or a bean bag to give the fetus as much room as possible in the pelvis. Your partner can help by massaging your back.*

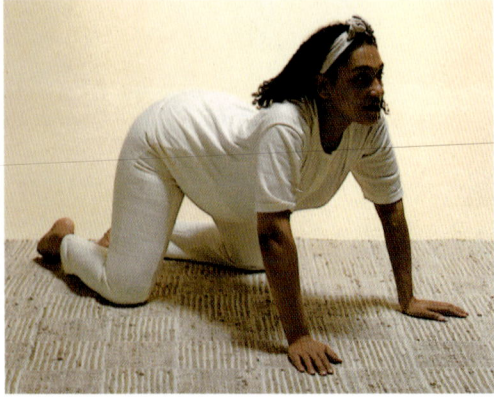

2 *Take the weight of the baby off your spine by kneeling on the floor on all fours with your arms and legs wide apart. Keep the small of your back flat and not hollowed.*

WEEK 32: POSITIONS FOR LABOUR

Your growing baby

The fetus is now very energetic and it will have periods of extreme activity, and you will feel it twisting and turning. As it continues to grow it will have less and less room to move in, so it will soon settle, probably in the head-down position, ready for birth. The fetus is about 40.5 cm/16 in long and weighs about 1.6 kg/3½ lb.

Partner support

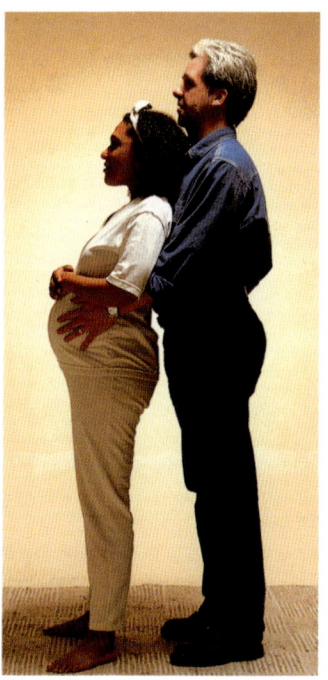

which you will need to relax. Kneeling with your legs wide apart and supported on both sides is another good position for pushing.

Once you have tried these positions, experiment with others which you feel may be right for you during labour. Try them on the floor, on the bed, leaning on or against furniture, or using your partner for support. This way, when you are in labour, you will already know how to get into positions that are comfortable for you and that will help you cope with contractions.

1 *Practise using your partner for support during labour by leaning back against him, allowing him to take your weight.*

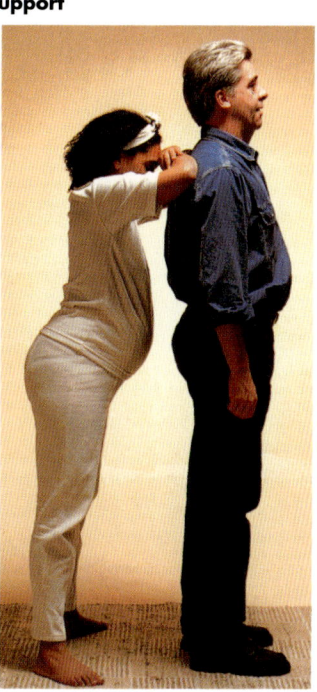

2 *Stand with feet well apart and lean on your partner, putting your head on your arms to ease pressure on your uterus.*

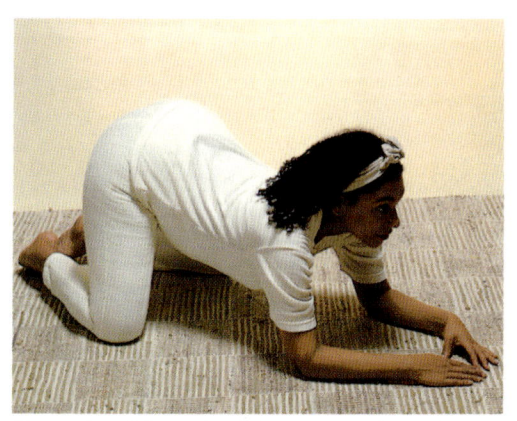

3 *Kneel on all fours with your forearms on the floor and your knees spread wide so that your abdomen is hanging between them. It can help to rock backwards and forwards in this position.*

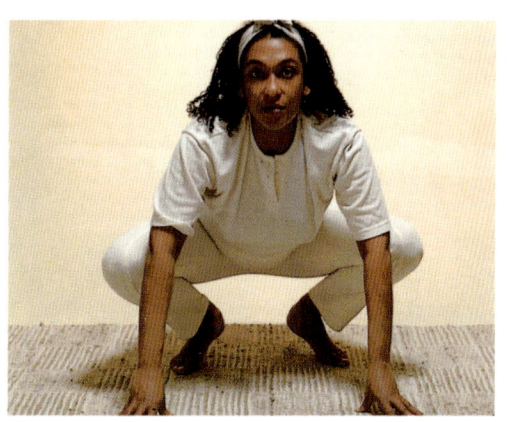

4 *In this squatting position, your pelvis is wide open and the baby's head is pressed down. You may find that it helps to place your hands on the floor to give yourself some support.*

WEEK 33: EMOTIONS IN LATE PREGNANCY

It is not just your body that is going through great changes while you are pregnant. Your whole way of life is changing and this can lead to conflicting emotions, especially during the last few months. You may wonder how you are going to cope with all the new responsibilities and be concerned about your baby – whether it will be born perfect in every way. Vivid dreams are common at this time and can be worrying, especially if they are about the birth or babies. You may even feel occasionally that the whole thing has been a ghastly mistake and that you want to go back to the way things were before you became pregnant. Don't worry, all these feelings are quite normal.

It helps to talk about your fears and concerns, either to your partner or to a close friend who has had similar feelings. Parentcraft classes are also a good place to discuss these worries, especially as you will be with other women who are experiencing the same emotions. If you find that talking about it doesn't help and that anxiety is taking over your life, discuss how you feel with your midwife or doctor.

Your partner

It is easy to forget that an expectant father is also going through emotional changes as he comes to terms with impending parenthood. He doesn't have any outward sign of the change that is about to occur in his life, but that doesn't mean he isn't feeling the same concerns as you. He also has additional worries about you and how you will cope during labour; he may even secretly fear for your safety during the birth. If he is now solely responsible for providing financially for you and the baby he may be feeling considerable stress.

Make time to talk to each other about your feelings and try to ensure that these last weeks before the birth are special for you both. Share the preparation for the birth so that each of you is involved in what is going to happen. Plan some treats where you can be alone together, such as a special dinner at a favourite restaurant, a trip to the theatre, or a weekend away at a hotel. By making time for yourselves you are less likely to have misunderstandings which could lead to hurt and disappointment.

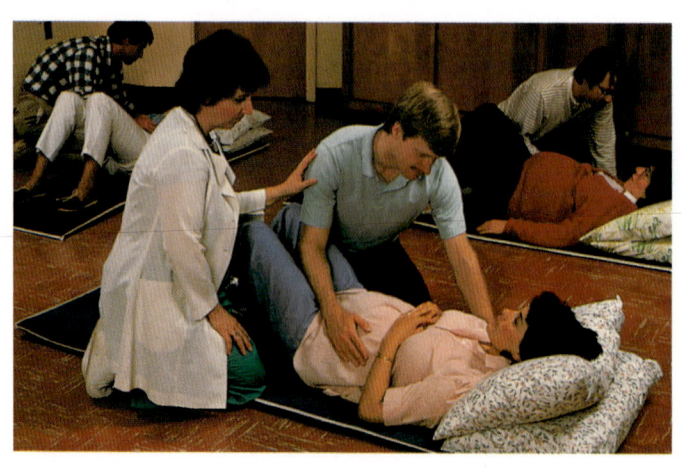

You and your body
Your weight gain should have slowed down. If it hasn't and you are still gaining more than 1 kg/2¼ lb a week, you should check with your doctor that everything is all right.

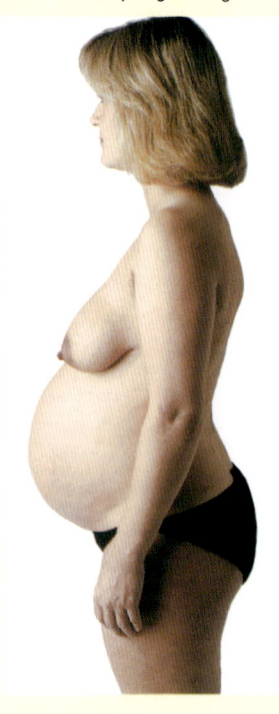

At ante-natal classes you learn what to expect in labour and the different positions you can adopt. Your partner is usually welcome to come with you and find out how he can help.

WEEK 33: EMOTIONS IN LATE PREGNANCY

Your growing baby

The fingernails are fully formed although the toenails are not quite so advanced. The vernix covering the skin has become thicker. The lungs are almost fully developed and the fetus will be practising breathing in preparation for the birth. It measures around 41.5 cm/16½ in and weighs about 1.8 kg/4 lb.

OTHER CHILDREN

If you have other children you may have told them about the new baby early on in your pregnancy. Very young children will need to have it explained to them over and over again, because the concept of a new baby is hard for them to grasp. Older children will probably be very excited and will enjoy being involved in any preparations you are making for their brother or sister.

How children react once the baby has arrived depends a lot on their age and personality, as well as their relationship with you. A preschool child may react by being naughty for a period in an attempt to get your attention. A toddler, who has recently been potty-trained, may start wetting or dirtying him- or herself again. Both age groups may start waking at night. Use common sense and tact to minimize any problems. Talk to your children about the new baby, encourage their help and involvement when he or she is born but always make sure that they have time with you on their own.

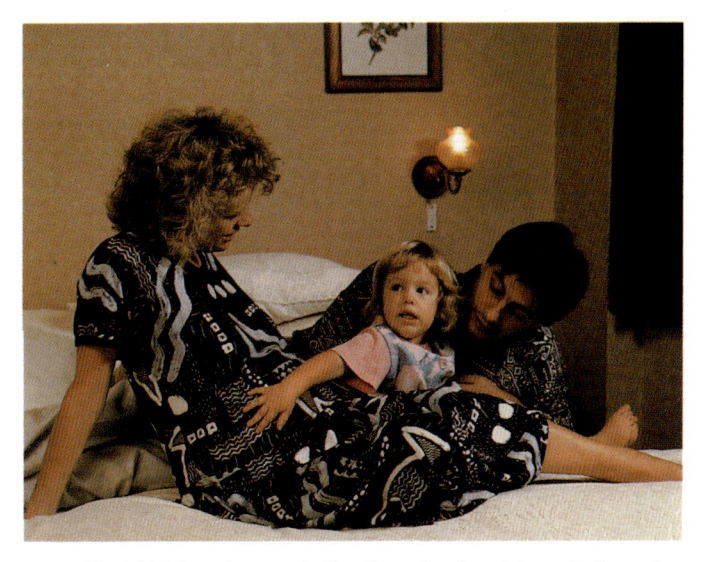

Let an older child feel your bump, and talk to him or her about their new brother or sister, so they can get used to the idea of a new family member.

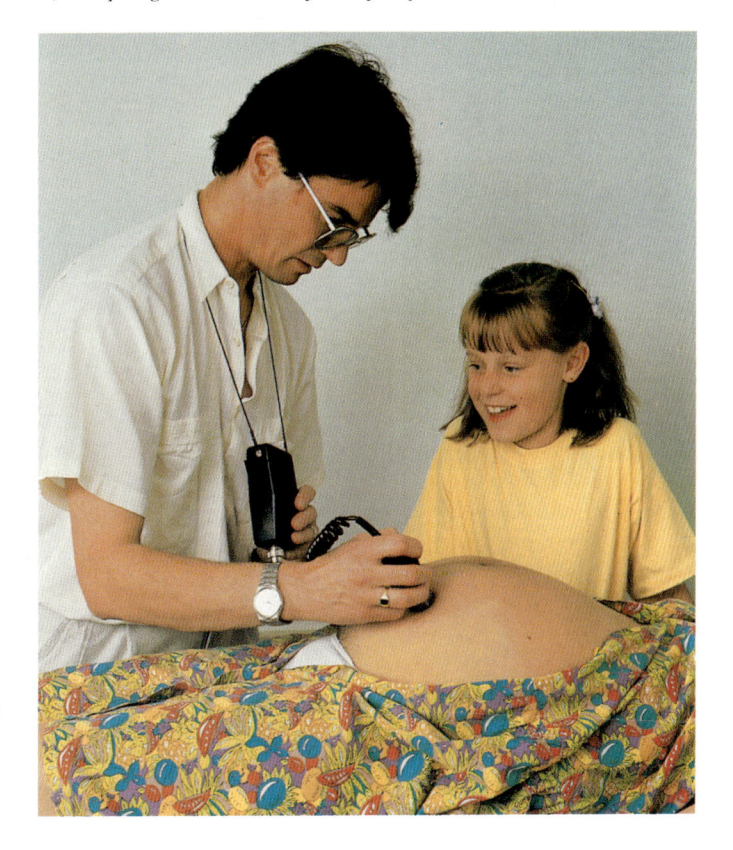

When your doctor checks your baby's heartbeat, let any older children be present if they are interested.

WEEK 34: OLDER FIRST-TIME MOTHERS

If you are 35 or over, you will have been offered an amniocentesis because of the higher risk of fetal abnormality. The amniotic fluid will have been screened for a number of chromosomal disorders, which include Down's syndrome and spina bifida. Of course, you don't have to have this test, but many mothers find it reassuring.

It is important that you attend all your ante-natal clinics so that a close check can be kept on you and the unborn baby all through pregnancy. Many older expectant mothers prefer to have the ante-natal care at a hospital where expert medical help is on hand. The risk to the baby during labour and birth increases with rising maternal age, but many factors affect labour, including the general health of the mother during pregnancy. Although nearly 70 per cent of women over 30 have normal deliveries, there is a greater risk of complications during labour for women who are over 35. This is usually because the baby is in distress through lack of oxygen because of placental deterioration. As a result of these complications older women tend to have more forceps and Caesarean deliveries.

BIRTH AND THE OLDER MOTHER
Most older women go full term, and if you are between 30 and 34 there is no reason why you shouldn't have a natural birth. If you are 35 or over, or if there is a suggestion that your baby may be small, you may have to have continuous monitoring. This may also be necessary if there is a likelihood of a prolonged labour, or if the waters, when they break, show some sign of staining. This means that you will be unable to move around freely. But this is a small

You and your body
Your blood pressure may be slightly raised and you will probably be told to take things easy. Swelling of the hands and feet could also be a problem so try to get as much rest as possible, preferably with your feet up.

Seeing her baby on an ultrasound scan can be very reassuring for an older mother.

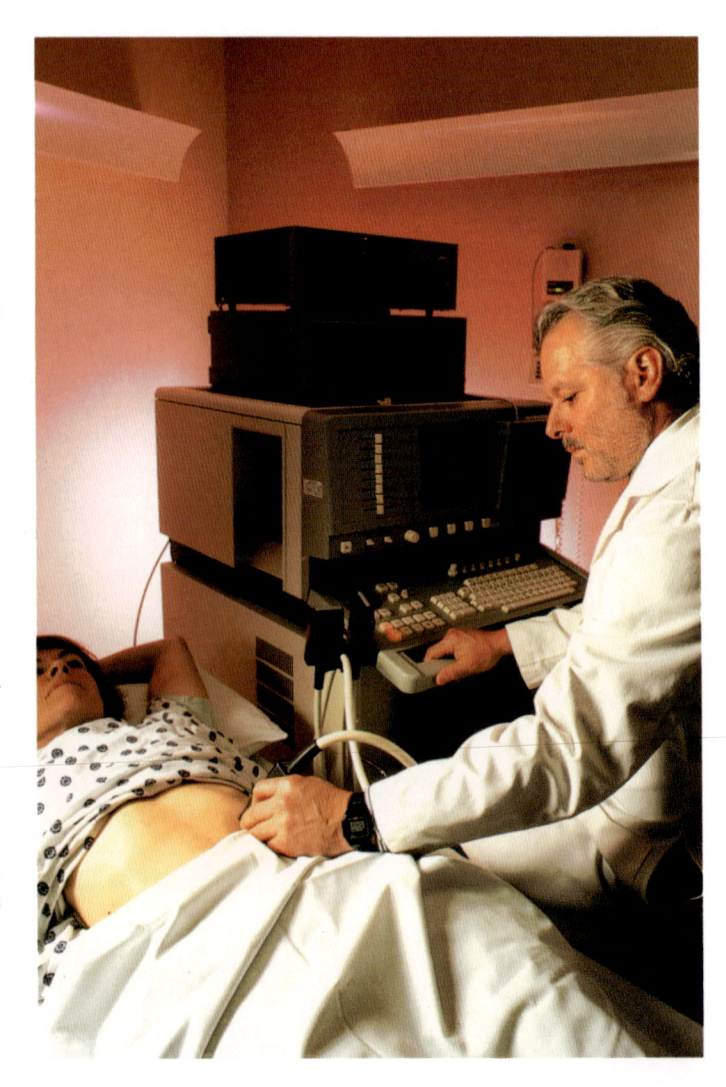

Week 34: Older First-time Mothers

price to pay for a healthy baby.

Babies born to older mothers have a greater chance of being born preterm. This is often because of the failure of the placenta, which means the baby is no longer getting sufficient oxygen and nourishment. If this happens you will probably have to have a forceps delivery, or you may be offered a Caesarean.

Your growing baby
The weight gain continues to increase. The eyes respond to bright lights and the fetus will practise blinking; eyebrows and eyelashes are fully developed. A boy's testicles will have descended into the groin. The fetus is 43 cm/17 in long and weighs about 2 kg/4½ lb.

Below: The doctor will talk about your baby and give you a printout of your scan.

Right: As time progresses, you will find you need more rest with your back supported.

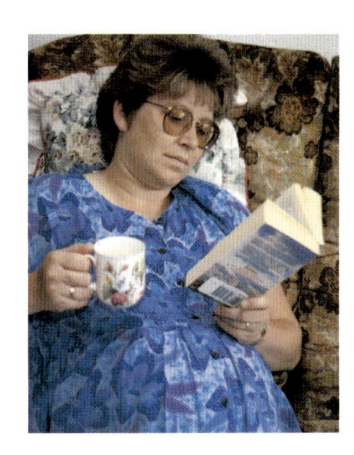

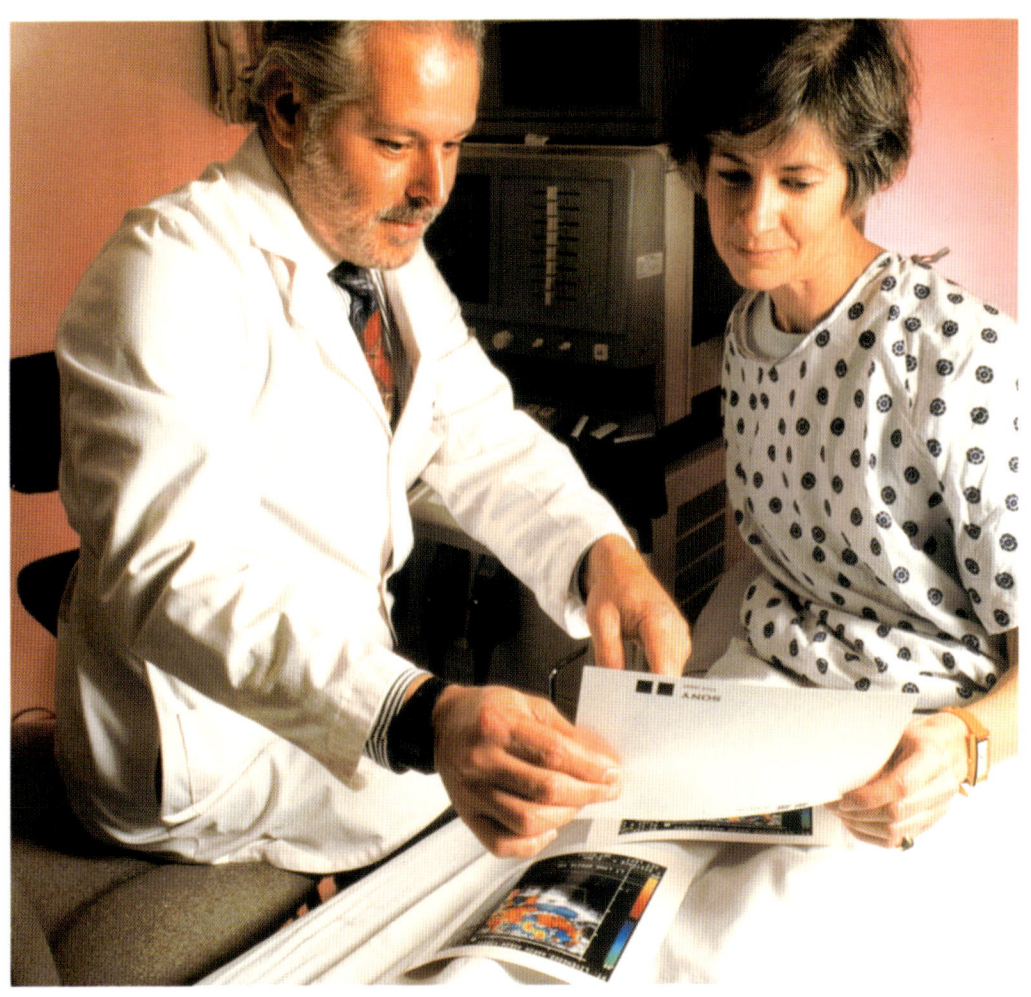

WEEK 35: FINAL PREPARATIONS

Even though your baby is not due for some weeks, you should be ready in case he or she decides to put in an early appearance. Check the nursery and make sure all the baby's sheets and blankets have been washed and aired. Sort out all the baby clothes and put the ones you will want immediately after the birth in your hospital case.

It's a good idea to stock up on non-perishable goods and to fill the freezer, if you have one. This will save you from having to do a lot of shopping over the next few weeks and will allow you more time with the baby when you first come home.

Make sure you know where your partner is going to be over the next few weeks; if he is out and about you may want to consider hiring a bleeper so that you can keep in constant touch. Keep your car filled with petrol and make sure that you both know the quickest route to the hospital. Have a list of emergency numbers, including a local taxi firm, beside the telephone.

THE HOSPITAL

Pack what you want to take to hospital several weeks before the delivery date; keep the bag where you can easily get it when the time comes. Remember that there are three separate aspects to consider: labour, your hospital stay, and going-home clothes for you and the baby.

You should bring any personal items that will make life more comfortable for you during labour. Include anything from a personal stereo and your favourite music to a face cloth and massage oils. You may even want to take along a bean bag if you are planning an active labour and your hospital doesn't provide these. Leave some room for last-minute items such as an ice pack for backache and even a snack and drink for your partner. Don't forget to put your birthplan and maternity record right at the top so that you can give these to the midwife when you

You and your body

Discuss any worries you may have about labour and birth with your doctor or midwife. You will be feeling tired and even a little fed up, so try to get as much rest as you can. Pay special attention to your diet: you will be needing another 200 calories a day during these last weeks. Some practical planning now can save time and forestall anxiety at the time of labour and delivery.

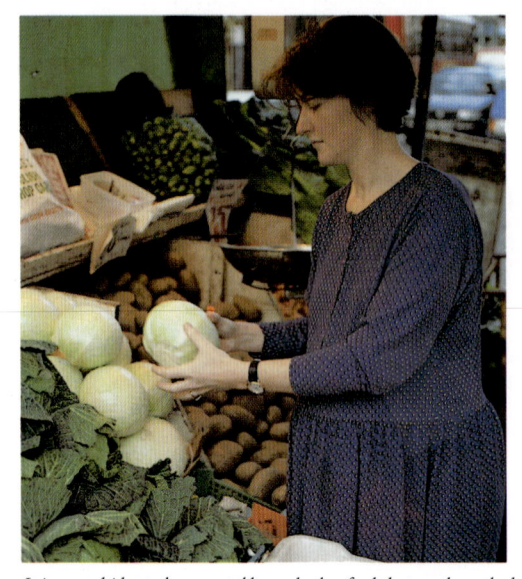

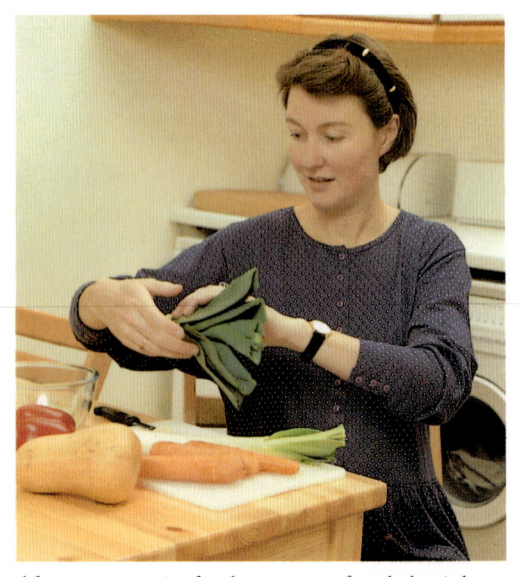

It is a good idea to buy vegetables and other food that can be cooked and frozen in preparation for when you return from the hospital.

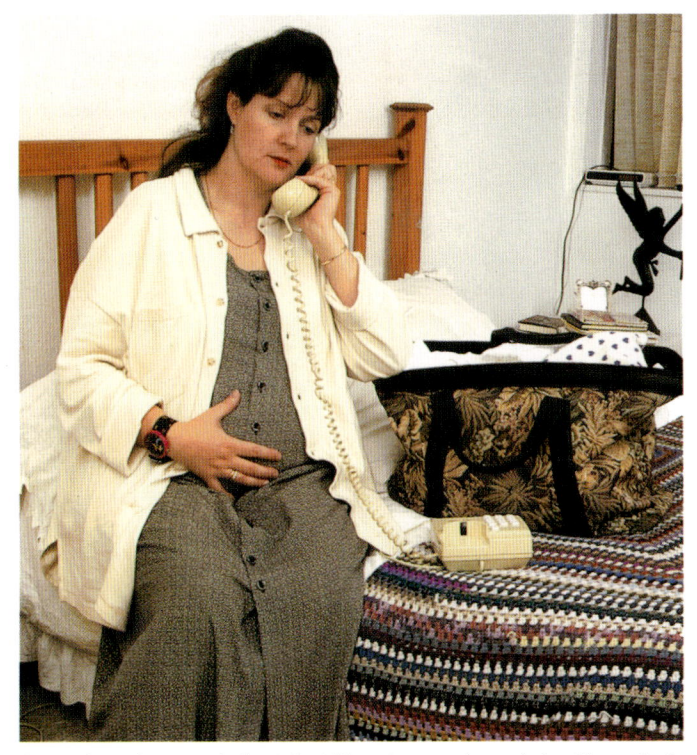

Week 35: Final Preparations

arrive at the hospital. It is sensible to pack things for labour separately, since you will want to be able to get to them quickly.

How much you pack for the hospital depends on your planned length of stay after the birth. The hospital may issue a list of the items that you will need to bring with you. But if it doesn't, ask your midwife whether you need to take in baby clothes and nappies, or contact the maternity unit direct. If you are staying in for a few days and aren't too tired, you might want to write cards to your friends and relatives announcing your baby's arrival, so remember to include birth announcement cards, your address book, and stamps. You should also bring change in case you need to use hospital pay phones.

You will need clothes for you and the baby when it's time for you to return home. It is sensible to pack a small bag now with all the items you think you'll want for your return journey; you can either bring it with you or your partner can bring it later. Remember that although you will feel considerably slimmer than you were before the birth, it takes a while before you get your figure back, so your going-home outfit will still need to be loose.

You might need to get to the hospital quickly, so have your bag packed and keep a local taxi number close to hand.

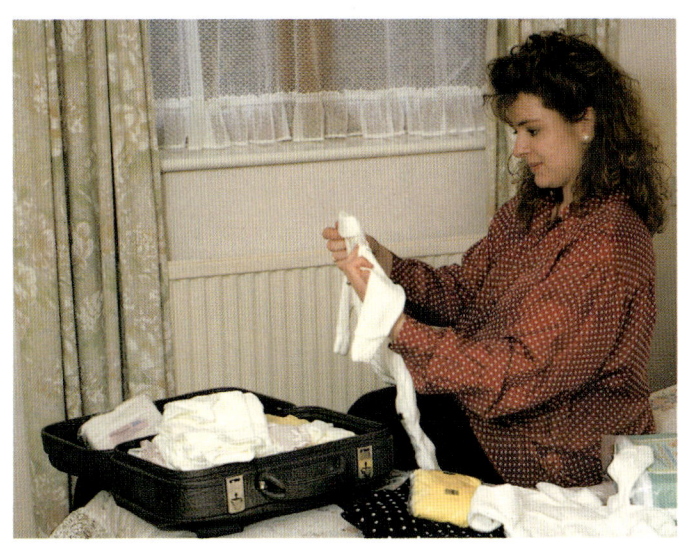

It is sensible to pack a small bag for your brief stay in hospital well in advance in case you have to leave in a rush. Don't forget some clothes for your new baby to wear.

Your growing baby

The fetus is putting on weight each day and now fills most of the uterus, so you may find it uncomfortable when it moves around. The fetus now does body rolls rather than the more energetic movements it made when it was smaller. It is now about 44.5 cm/ 17½ in long and weighs around 2.3 kg/5 lb.

WEEK 36: DISCOMFORTS IN LATE PREGNANCY

You and your body
You will be able to feel the top of your uterus just below your breastbone. This can make breathing uncomfortable and you may suffer from pain in your ribcage. Your ante-natal checks will be weekly from now on.

As you find getting around more difficult and everything generally more of an effort, you may become irritable over the smallest things. You will be impatient for your baby to arrive, and concern about the impending birth and worries about how you will cope with being a parent can make you short-tempered, especially with your partner. Tell him how you are feeling so that he understands why you are being so irritable and perhaps not paying him as much attention as usual.

Aches or pains around your pubic area, in your groin, or down the inside of your legs can be caused by your baby's head pressing on the nerves, or by your pelvic joints beginning to soften in preparation for labour. Pain under your ribs is caused by the expanding uterus pushing the ribs up. These aches and pains are not serious, but they can be quite uncomfortable. Sitting or standing as straight as you can, or stretching upwards, will help ease most of these discomforts, although you may find lying down better for relief of pelvic pain. If you get severe pain in your abdomen, or if you suffer any abdominal pain that is also accompanied by vaginal bleeding, you must get in touch with your doctor at once.

It is quite common to suffer from heartburn and nausea towards the end of pregnancy. This is caused by the enlarged uterus pressing on your stomach. It often helps to eat small

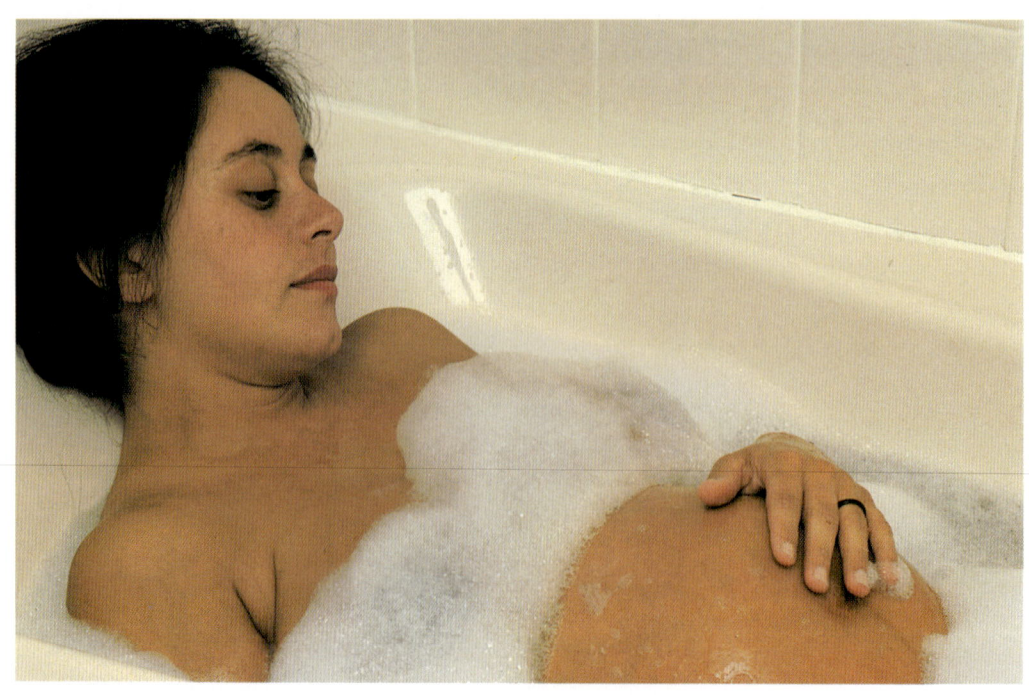

Soaking in a warm bath can help to relieve any aches and pains you are suffering.

Week 36: Discomforts in Late Pregnancy

meals at frequent intervals, rather than two or three big meals a day.

Ante-natal check

An internal examination or a scan may be carried out to check the size of your pelvis. If there is any concern about the size of your pelvis in relation to your baby's size, or there is some other reason for the baby's delivery not being straightforward, a Caesarean may be discussed. If this is thought to be necessary, the doctor at the hospital where the delivery is to take place will explain the medical procedures that will be used.

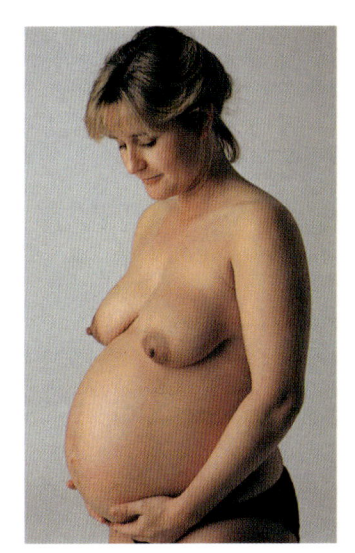

As your baby increases in size, you may begin to find breathing uncomfortable and get some pain in your ribcage.

Your growing baby

The nervous system is maturing and the fetus is getting ready for birth by starting to practise breathing movements, sucking, and swallowing. It is now about 46 cm/18¼ in long and weighs around 2.5 kg/5½ lb.

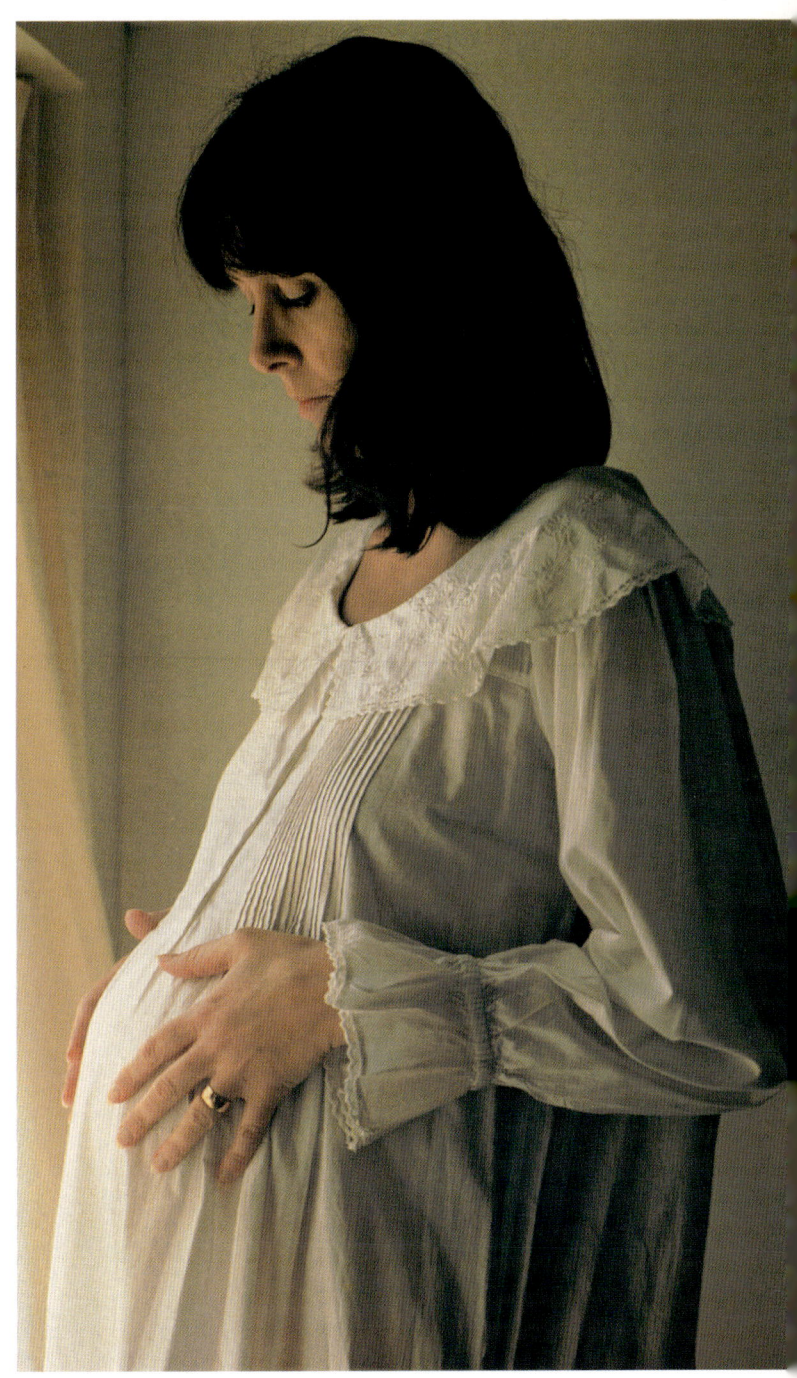

In this late stage of pregnancy you will probably be able to feel the top of your uterus which is now positioned just below your breastbone.

WEEK 37: AS BIRTH APPROACHES

Your growing baby
The lanugo, the fine hair that covers the fetus's body, is beginning to wear off. The fetus has started to produce a hormone called cortisone which will help the lungs to become fully matured so that they are ready to cope with breathing once it is born. The fetus will be practising breathing although there is no air in its lungs. The fetus is now about 47cm/18½ in long and weighs around 2.7 kg/6 lb.

Between weeks 36 and 38 the baby's head is likely to "engage". This is when it settles downwards, deep in your pelvis ready for the birth. You should feel some relief from the pressure in your abdomen when this happens which is why it is sometimes referred to as "lightening". You will start to feel less breathless now because the baby is no longer putting any pressure on your diaphragm and your lungs.

If this is not your first baby, but your second or third child, the head may not engage until you actually go into labour.

PREMATURE AND TWIN BIRTHS
If the baby is born before 37 weeks it will be described as being preterm or premature. Most premature babies are nursed in a special care baby unit (SCBU) or, if very sick or small, an intensive care baby unit (ICBU). Babies are given expert care and

This is probably the last time for a while that you will have time to yourself, so make the most of it and rest often.

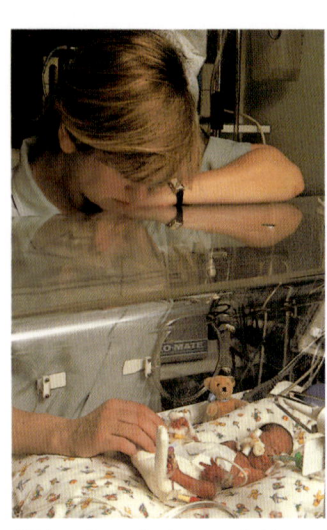

With modern technology even babies as young as 24 weeks normally survive in the special baby units.

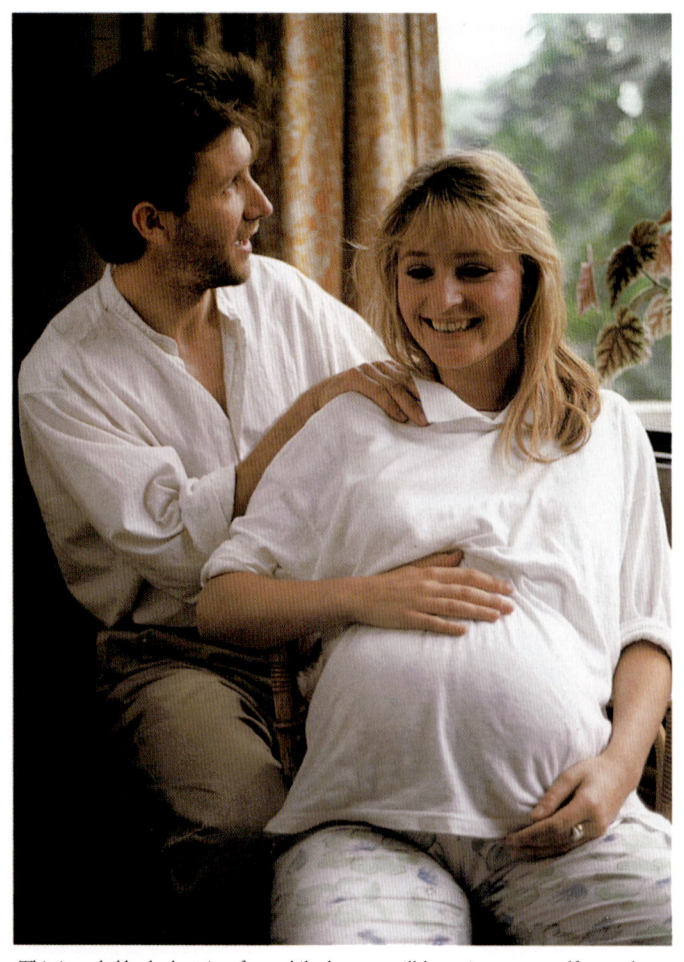

Week 37: As Birth Approaches

attention in these facilities, so that even those who are born as young as 24 weeks have a reasonable chance of survival.

If you are giving birth to twins, the labour doesn't usually take any longer than if you are giving birth to a single baby (singleton). Because twins tend to be smaller babies, the labour and birth can often be easier and less painful. Once the birth canal has been stretched to allow one baby to be born, the second baby will usually be born quite quickly. If twins share the placenta, they will both be born before it is delivered. Even if they are fraternal twins and each have their own placenta they will usually be born first, although occasionally one baby is born, followed by its placenta, before the second baby arrives.

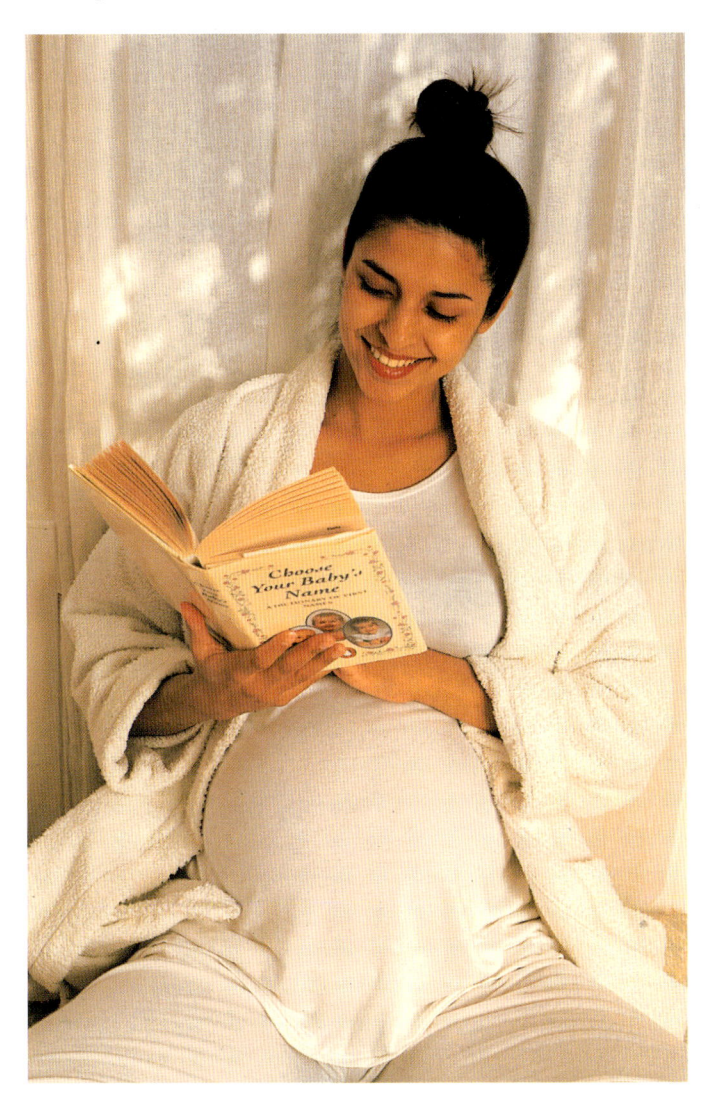

You and your body

Your baby could arrive at any time from now until the end of week 42, so check that you have everything organized. You will probably be able to visit the hospital about now and see where you are going to give birth. Don't be afraid to ask questions if there is anything you don't understand about hospital procedures.

Sometime between now and the birth, you may experience a sudden burst of energy, known as the nesting instinct. Don't overdo things and decide to spring-clean your whole house. Remember that you will shortly need all your energy reserves for the exhausting demands of labour.

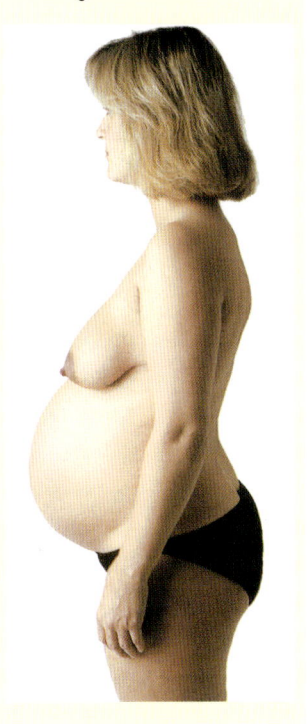

As the birth approaches, it is a good time for you and your partner to start making a list of names that you both like.

WEEK 38: INDUCTION/PAIN RELIEF IN LABOUR

You and your body
You will notice that the fetus is moving about less now that it is head down in the uterus. You may be feeling tired and rather depressed about the waiting so try to keep busy.

Sometimes labour has to be started artificially because of a problem such as pre-eclampsia, bleeding, diabetes, or you are well past your due date and the placenta is no longer working efficiently. Induction involves several techniques.

Pessaries Prostaglandin pessaries, made from a naturally occurring hormone, may be inserted into the vagina to soften the cervix and to start the contractions.

Artificial rupture of the membranes (ARM) This involves puncturing the amniotic sac in which the baby is sealed so that the increased pressure on the cervix causes the contractions to become much stronger.

Syntocinon drip A hormone that stimulates contractions is put into a vein to help them remain constant and steady. This may lead to stronger contractions than you would otherwise have had.

PAIN RELIEF
You will have been told about the various forms of pain relief at parentcraft classes. If you want to have a completely natural birth make sure that this is marked clearly on your birthplan and inform the medical staff who will be attending you during labour.

Remember that you can always change your mind later if you find coping with the pain too difficult. If you have decided to opt for some form of pain relief, there are a number of options you can choose from:

Gas and air (Entonox) A mixture of oxygen and nitrous oxide which is breathed in through a mask and takes the edge off pain. This is the most controllable form of pain relief because you hold the mask and regulate the gas and air intake yourself. The gas is processed in your lungs so it doesn't affect the baby.

Injections Drugs like pethidine and meptid can be given during the first stage of labour. They will help you relax and relieve pain but they can affect the baby, making him sleepy at birth and afterwards.

Epidural A local anaesthetic is injected into the space between your spinal column and the spinal cord, numbing the nerves that serve the uterus. It may also numb your leg nerves, making it hard for you to move around. An epidural may also be used if a Caesarean delivery is performed because it allows the mother to stay awake while her baby is being delivered.

An anaesthetist is needed to give an epidural injection, which takes around 30 minutes to set up, and then usually requires topping up every hour and a half.

Transcutaneous electrical nerve stimulation (TENS) This is a technique which involves a weak electric current being used to block pain sensations in the brain and to

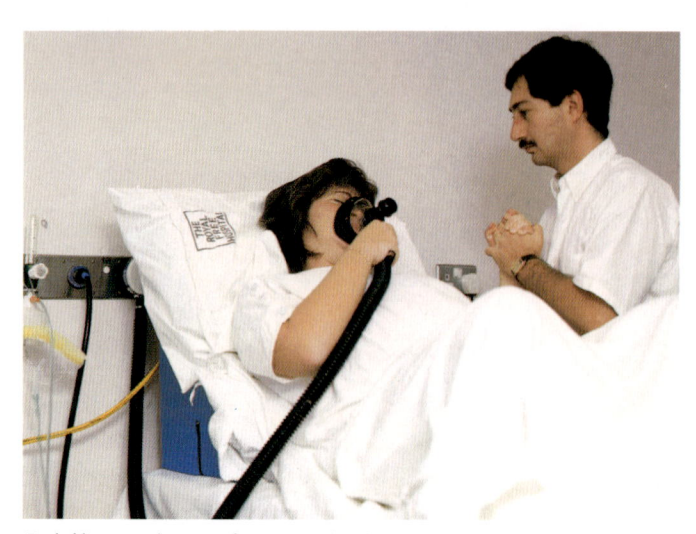

By holding a mask to your face, you can breathe in oxygen and nitrous oxide for pain relief during contractions.

WEEK 38: INDUCTION/PAIN RELIEF IN LABOUR

stimulate the release of endorphins, the body's natural painkilling hormones. TENS is not available at all hospitals so you may need to hire a machine before you go into labour.

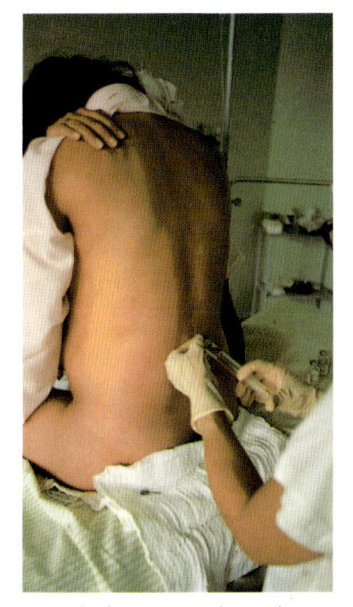

An epidural injection into the spinal area helps deaden the nerves around the uterus.

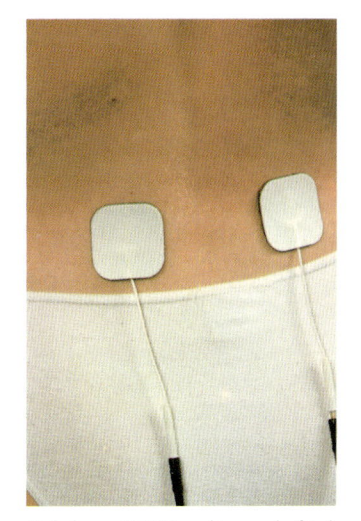

Pads from a TENS machine can be fitted to your back to ease pain in labour.

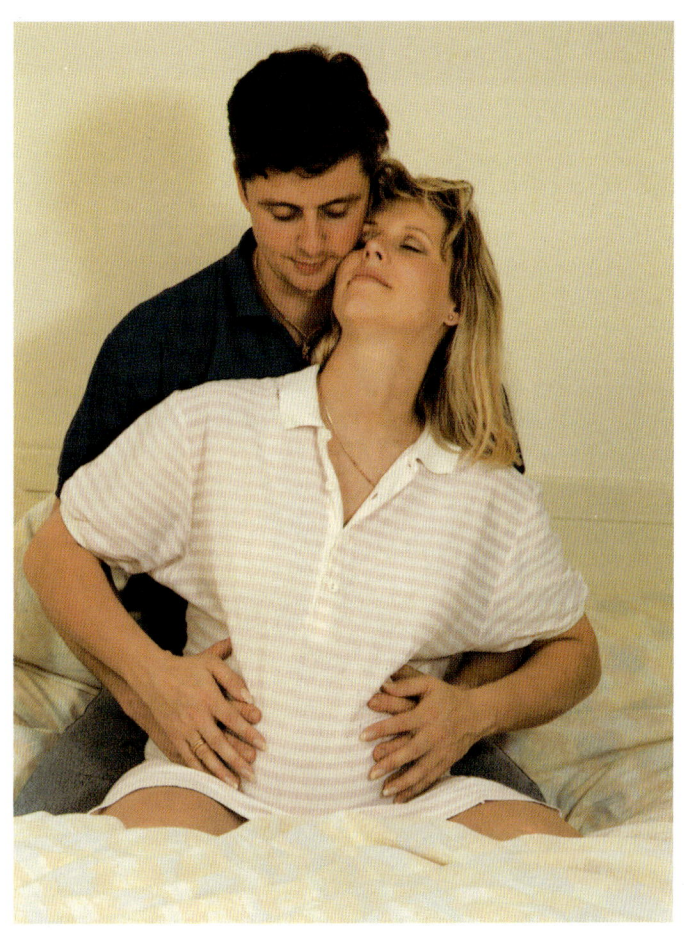

At the most painful times in your labour, lean on your partner for support and encouragement. He can also massage your back if it is really painful.

Your midwife should be able to give you all the necessary details.

Alternative pain relief Both acupuncture and hypnosis can be used to relieve pain during childbirth, but if you are having a hospital birth you will need permission to have a private practitioner with you during labour. Used correctly, massage, aromatherapy, and reflexology can all help to ease labour. You should get some expert advice before the birth if you intend to use any of these techniques.

Your growing baby

The fetus has put on fat so that it now appears rounded and its skin has a pinkish look. The hair may be as long as 5 cm/2 in and the nails already need cutting. The vernix, which has been protecting the skin of the growing fetus from the amniotic fluid, is beginning to dissolve. At this stage of your pregnancy, the fetus now measures about 48 cm/19 in and weighs around 2.9 kg/6½ lb.

WEEK 39: COMPLICATIONS DURING BIRTH

The ideal position for your baby to be born is with its head lying down with its back against your abdomen. This way it has less distance to rotate in the birth canal. Sometimes a baby is in an abnormal position which can make birth more complicated, but this does not necessarily mean that it can't be born in the normal way.

An occipito posterior position means that the baby is lying with its back towards your back and, if it fails to turn, will be delivered normally, but will be born face up. This way of lying often leads to a long, back-aching labour.

In a deep transverse arrest, the baby's head partially rotates in the birth canal and then becomes stuck with its face towards one side. The baby will need to be helped out. This can sometimes also happen if you push too hard by mistake in the second stage of labour.

Disproportion means that the baby's head is too big for your pelvis. A scan will be done to decide whether there is enough room for a normal delivery to take place. If there isn't, your baby will probably be born by Caesarean.

Breech birth

A small number of babies don't turn around in the last weeks of pregnancy. This means that their feet or bottom would come out first so the birth canal will not have been stretched enough when the head, the largest part of the baby's body, is ready to be born. Doctors have different opinions about the best way of delivering a breech baby; some insist that a Caesarean is the safest method, others believe that birth should take place under an epidural, and some think that if the mother remains mobile throughout the first stage of labour the baby will get itself into a good position for birth. It may then be helped out with forceps or by vacuum extraction.

Birth positions

A normal birth

A breech birth

You and your body

The waiting is nearly over and you will probably be feeling both excited and apprehensive. You may be having quite strong Braxton Hicks contractions as the cervix softens in readiness for the birth. Although you may be feeling heavy and weary, don't simply sit around waiting for something to happen. Keep up your social life and talk to other friends from your parent-craft classes who are at the same stage as you.

Forceps delivery

In a forceps delivery, your legs will be put up in stirrups and then the forceps, which are like a pair of large, shallow metal spoons, will be inserted into the vagina and cupped around the baby's head. The doctor helps the baby out while you push.

Vacuum extraction

Vacuum extraction (ventouse) is sometimes used instead of the forceps method. With this technique the doctor places a suction cup on the baby's head and the baby is sucked out as you push down with each contraction.

If the birth canal is not going to be big enough for the baby's head and there is a risk that the perineum may tear, a small cut is made in this area under local anaesthetic. This

Your growing baby

The fetus is now able to function on its own, although it is still getting nourishment from the placenta. The fetus is in position for birth and is about 49 cm/ 19¼ in long and weighs around 3.1 kg/7 lb.

WEEK 39: COMPLICATIONS DURING BIRTH

type of incision is called an episiotomy and is stitched after the birth, again under local anaesthetic.

FETAL MONITORING
This keeps a check on the unborn baby's heartbeat during labour and birth. Monitoring can be done the low-tech way by simply placing a stethoscope against the patient's abdomen, or through electronic fetal monitoring (EFM).

There are two types of EFM and they both give a continuous readout of the baby's heart and uterine contractions; if the EFM method is used then you are having a high-tech birth.

There are two different methods of fetal monitoring. The basic method is to listen to the fetal heartbeat using a fetal stethoscope (top right). The position of the baby will also be checked at the same time (right). Electronic fetal monitoring (EFM) (below) involves placing a belt around your bump which is attached to a monitor. This gives a continuous readout of the baby's heart.

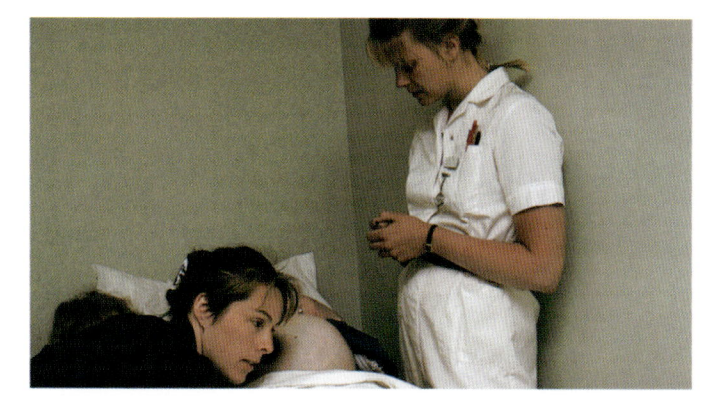

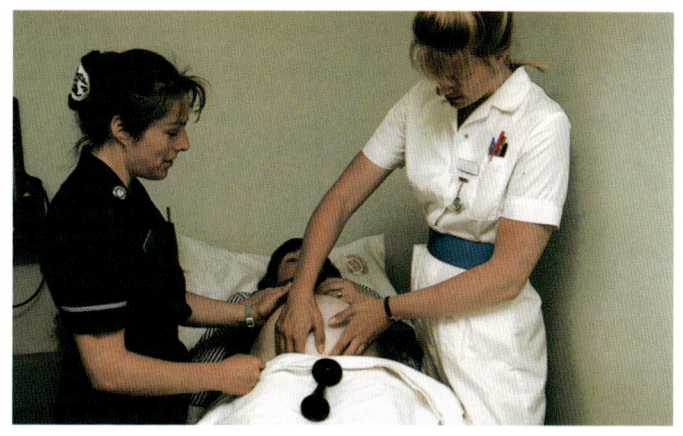

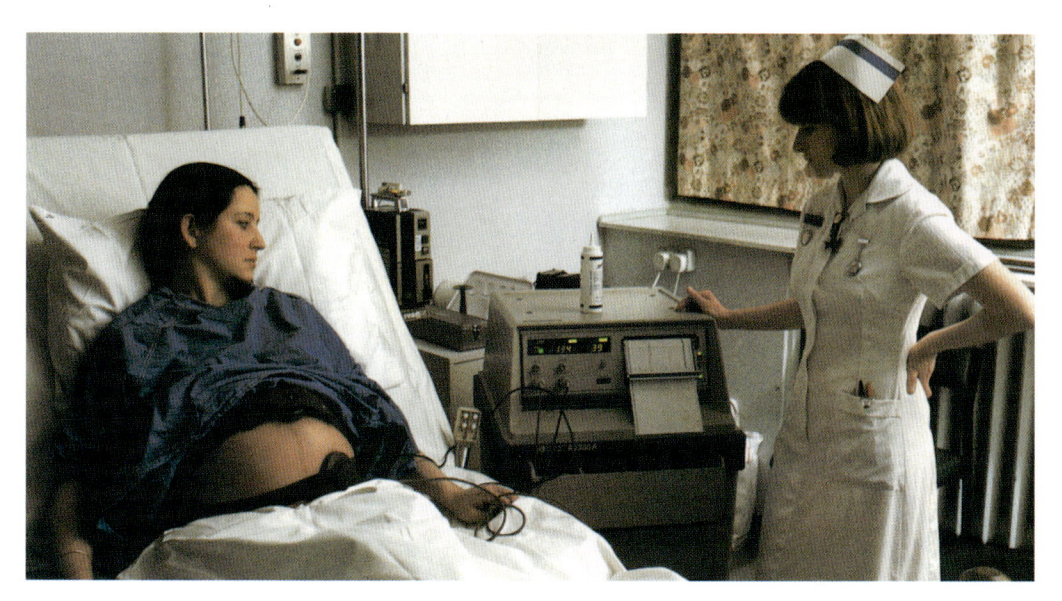

WEEK 40: LABOUR AND BIRTH

It is unlikely that you won't recognize the beginnings of labour as the signs, when they come, are generally unmistakable. There are three main indications that labour is about to start, or has started, and they can occur in any order. Once one or more of these has occurred you should let the hospital or midwife know immediately:

A show The protective plug, which sealed the cervix at the neck of the uterus, comes away and passes down the vagina. It usually appears as a small amount of bloodstained mucus. A show occurs before labour starts or during the first stage.

Waters breaking The membranes of the amniotic sac in which your baby has been floating break, causing either a trickle or a sudden gush of clear fluid from the vagina. If the fluid is yellow, greenish, or brown in colour you will need to go to the hospital straight away because the baby may be in distress. Your waters can break hours before labour starts or when it is well underway.

Contractions The regular tightening of the muscles of the uterus occurs throughout labour. During the first stage, the contractions thin out and dilate the cervix from closed to 10 cm/4 in open; in the second stage they help to push the baby down the vagina and after the birth they then deliver the placenta (afterbirth). For most women they feel rather like bad period pains. Contractions may also be accompanied by uncomfortable backache, sickness, and diarrhoea.

You and your body

You will probably be impatient for labour to start as you approach your EDD. If nothing has happened by your due date try not to be too disappointed; only around five per cent of babies actually arrive on the date they were expected. Keep yourself busy and make plans for each day so that you are not just sitting and waiting for something to happen. Once you are close to your EDD you may feel more confident wearing a sanitary towel just in case your waters break.

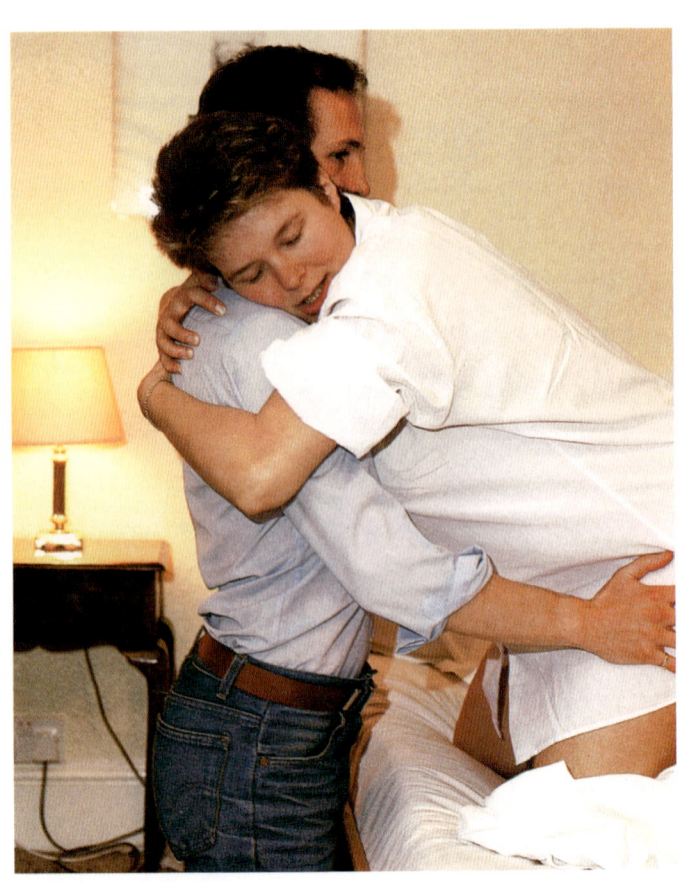

Your growing baby

Your baby is curled up, head down, in the fetal position with legs drawn up underneath and waiting to be born. He or she measures about 50 cm/19¾ in and weighs around 3.4 kg/7½ lb.

During the first stage of labour, you can involve your partner by leaning and holding onto him for comfort and also physical support.

Week 40: Labour and Birth

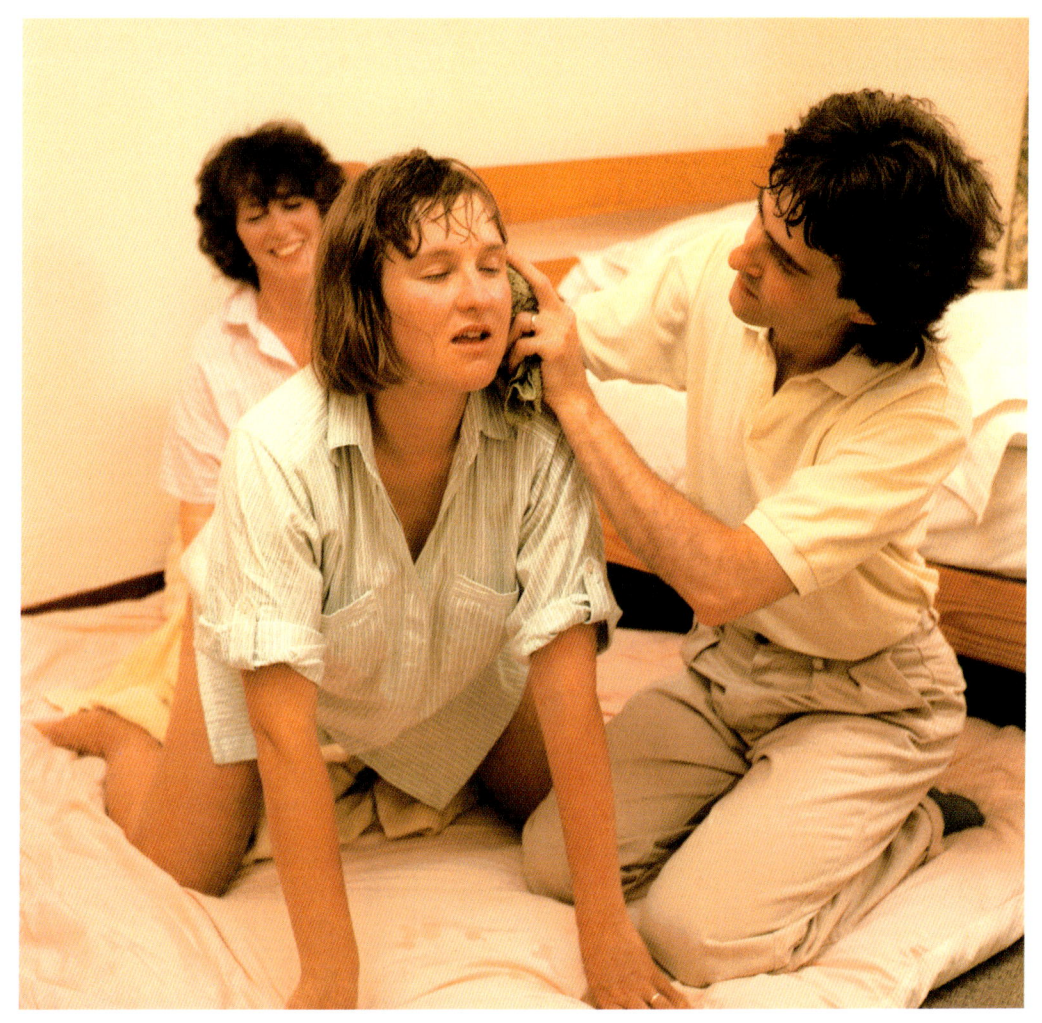

Your partner can help and encourage you when you're on all fours to keep the weight of the baby off your back in an active birth.

Stages of labour

The first stage: There are three stages of labour and the first is usually the longest, lasting generally from 12 hours upwards for a first baby. Contractions, which may have started off as mild and infrequent will, by the end of the first stage, be very strong and coming close together. Once they are coming regularly

Tips for labour

- Keep active for as long as you can during the first stage of labour.
- Don't be on your own: get your partner, mother or a friend to stay with you once labour has started.
- If your waters break check that the fluid is clear: yellow, greenish, or brown fluid could mean that your baby is in distress and you should go to the hospital immediately.
- Try different positions to help you cope with the pain of contractions.
- Ask for pain relief if you need it.
- Get your birth partner to make sure your wishes are known to whoever is delivering your baby. You may be too busy coping with contractions to explain clearly what you want.
- Put your baby to the breast soon after the birth. This will stimulate your milk supply and help to speed up the delivery of the placenta.

Week 40: Labour and Birth

every 10 minutes, or are each lasting for around 45 seconds, you should start getting ready to go to the hospital, or call the midwife if you are having your baby at home. When you get to the hospital, or the midwife attending you at home arrives, you will be examined to see how far your cervix has dilated and your blood pressure will be checked.

Although you will be able to carry on fairly normally for quite a lot of the first stage you should have someone with you. It is advisable to eat very little once labour has begun in case you need an emergency anaesthetic for any reason and to avoid being sick.

Towards the end of the first stage you will go into what is known as the transitional stage which can last for anything up to an hour. During this transitional period your baby moves down the birth canal and you will feel pressure on your back passage which may make you want to start pushing, even though the cervix is not fully dilated. By using the breathing techniques you have been taught you will be able to control this urge.

The second stage: Once the cervix is fully dilated and you start pushing the baby out you have entered the second stage. It can last for as little as half an hour or for as long as two hours or more. Once the baby's head is visible to the midwife she will tell you to start pushing. When the head reaches the vaginal opening you will be told to pant in short breaths so that the head can be delivered as slowly as possible. This allows the skin and muscle of the perineum to stretch so that the head can be born. If tearing seems likely an episiotomy, a small cut in the perineum, the area between the vagina and anus, may be given. Once the head is born your baby's body will follow quite quickly.

As soon as your baby is delivered it will be lifted onto your stomach for you to see it. The umbilical cord will be clamped and cut and the midwife will check the baby to make sure that it is all right and breathing properly. You may want to put your baby straight to the breast. You'll certainly wish to admire it with your partner and welcome your child into the world.

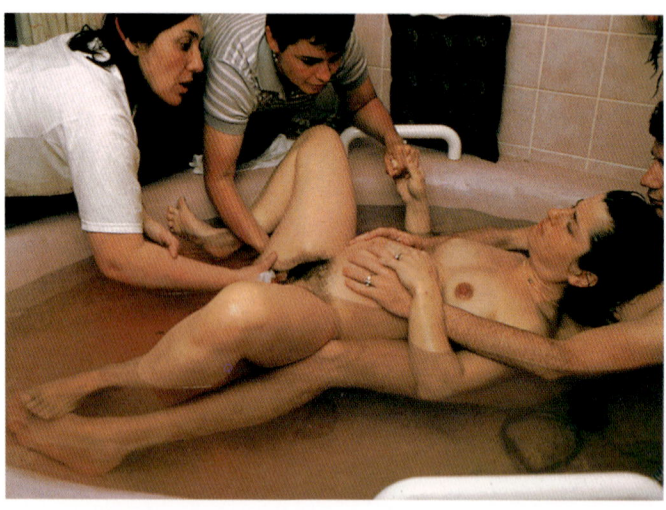

With a water birth, contractions can be eased by the warm water. Your baby can be delivered in the water or outside.

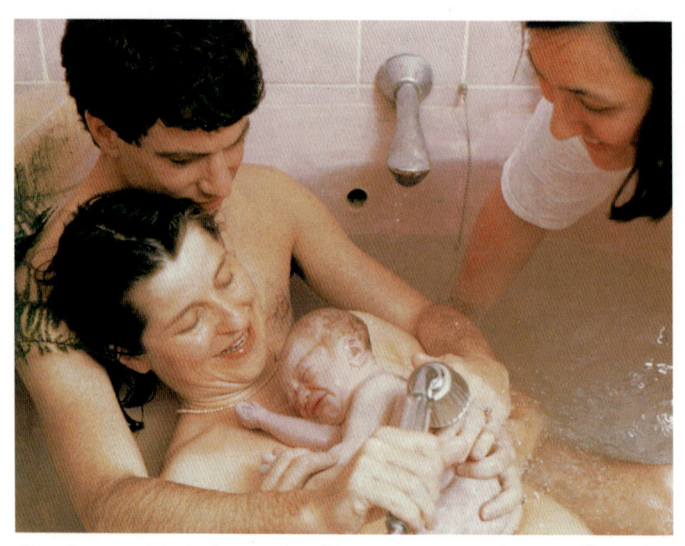

If you have your baby in the water, he will be given to you immediately after the birth for you and your partner to cuddle.

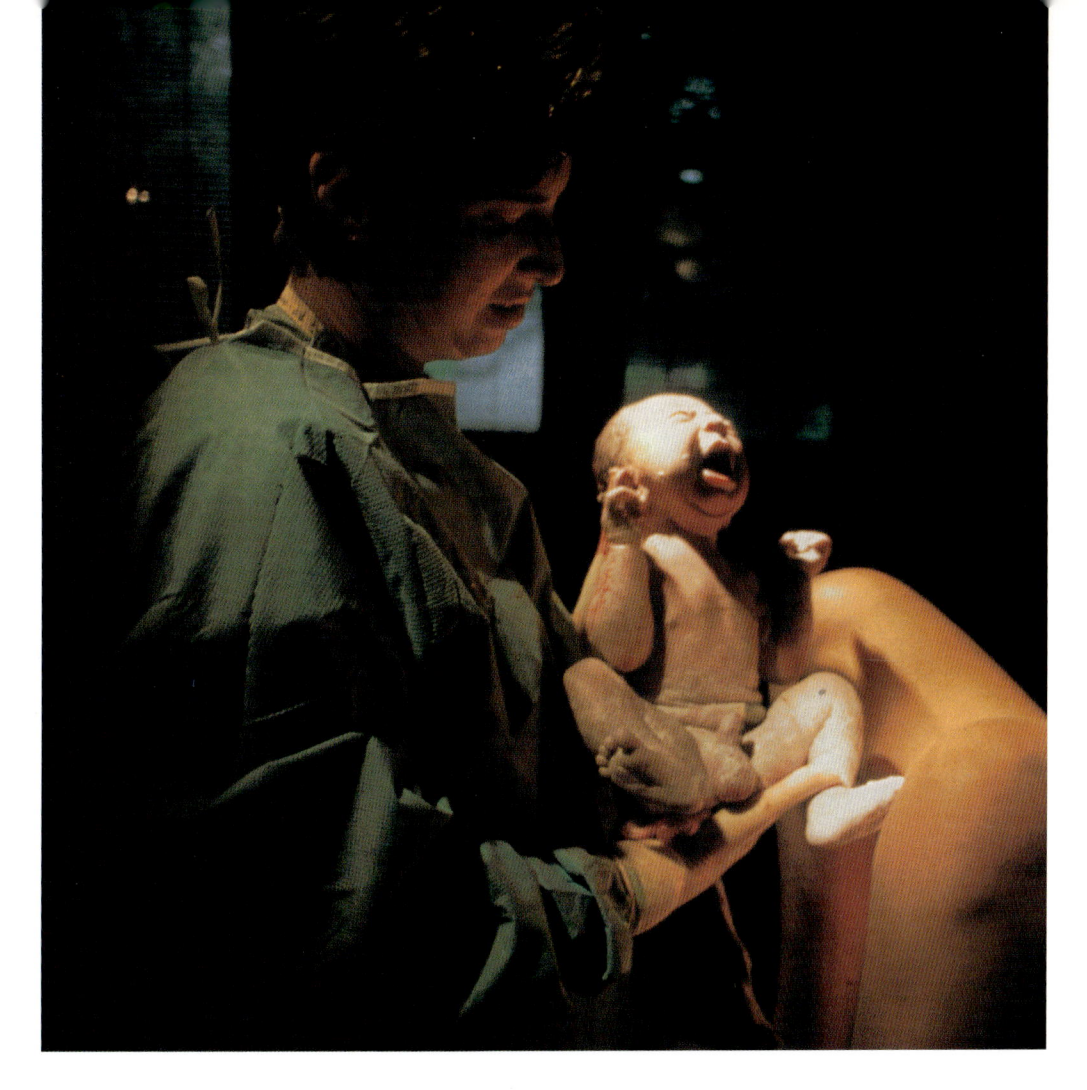

Above: A doctor holding a newborn baby boy, with the umbilical cord still attached, at a home delivery.
Right: With a Caesarean the baby is delivered through an incision. It is performed when there are risks from natural childbirth.

The third stage: The final stage of labour is the birth of the placenta, which usually takes less than half an hour. You may be given an injection to speed up the delivery. The midwife will check to see that the placenta is whole and that nothing has been left inside you. If you have had an episiotomy it will be stitched up.

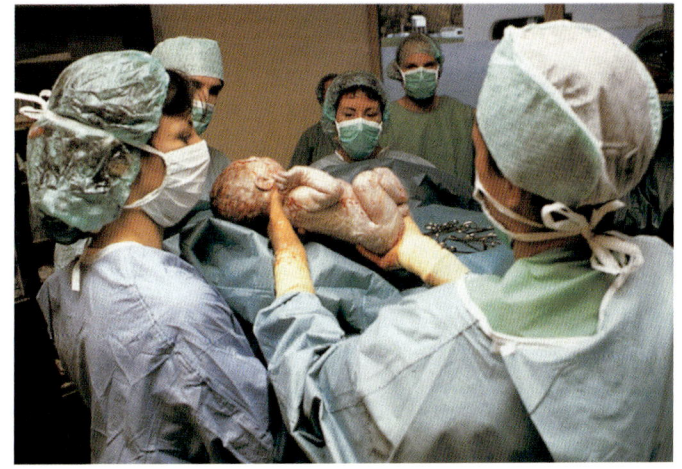

POST-NATAL CARE

Although your new baby will probably give you intense emotional satisfaction, you may well be physically uncomfortable. Your body has gone through many changes during pregnancy and it will take a while for it to return to its pre-pregnancy state.

Six weeks after the birth your doctor will examine you to make sure that everything is returning to normal; this also gives you a chance to discuss any worries you may have. The doctor will take your blood pressure and check a sample of your urine. Your breasts and abdomen will be examined and the doctor will make sure that any stitches have healed properly. You will probably have an internal examination to check the size and position of your uterus and you may have a cervical smear test if one is due.

If your baby was born in hospital, a midwife or doctor will probably talk to you about contraception before you go home. Alternatively, you can discuss this at your six-week check. Don't take any risks; to avoid getting pregnant again you should use contraception as soon as you resume intercourse. It is an old wives' tale that breast-feeding prevents conception.

If you were not immune to rubella (German measles) during your pregnancy, you will probably be offered the immunization before you leave hospital or at your six-week check-up. Ask your doctor if you are at all unsure about your immunity.

Your body

Immediately after the birth your breasts will produce colostrum, a high-protein liquid full of antibodies. Then, after the pregnancy hormones decline, your main milk supply should come in around the third or fourth day. At this time the breasts swell, feel hard, and can sometimes be painful. Bathing them with warm water is soothing, and letting the baby have frequent feeds will also help. This initial swelling subsides after a few days as both you and your baby get used to feeding. However, if you have decided to bottle-feed, your breasts will remain full for a few days until they gradually stop producing milk. Your breasts will probably never be quite as firm as they were before pregnancy, but a well-fitting support bra and exercise will help greatly.

After delivery your abdomen will probably be quite flabby and wrinkled because of slack muscles and stretched skin. Gentle post-natal exercises will help tighten up your abdominal and vaginal muscles, so make time to do them every day. If you feel you're not disciplined enough to exercise on your own, join a local post-natal class.

Following the birth you will have a vaginal discharge which is known as lochia. This will be like a very heavy period for a few days, with the flow gradually getting lighter until it disappears within a few weeks. Use maternity pads or large sanitary towels to absorb the discharge because there is a risk of infection if you use tampons in the early weeks after the birth. Your uterus will take about six weeks to

---

Your newborn will find your physical presence very reassuring during the first days after the birth. She will also find your smell comfortingly familiar.

Post-natal exercises

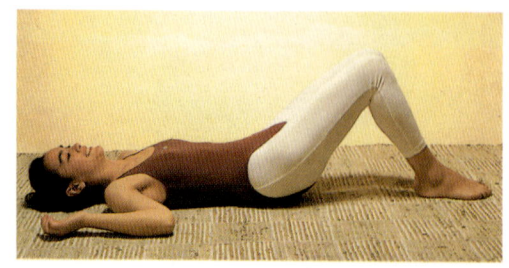

Pelvic floor: Lie flat on the floor with your legs drawn up and slightly apart. Close the back passage by drawing it in, hold for the count of four, then relax. Do as often as possible.

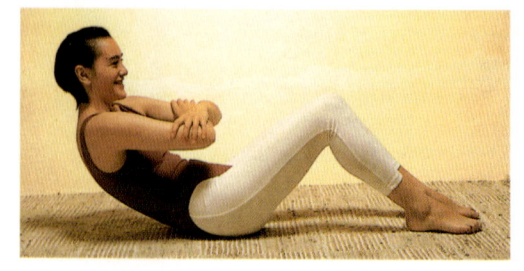

Tummy toner: Sit up with knees bent and feet flat on the floor. Fold arms in front. Lean back until you feel the abdominal muscles tighten, hold, then sit up and relax. Repeat several times.

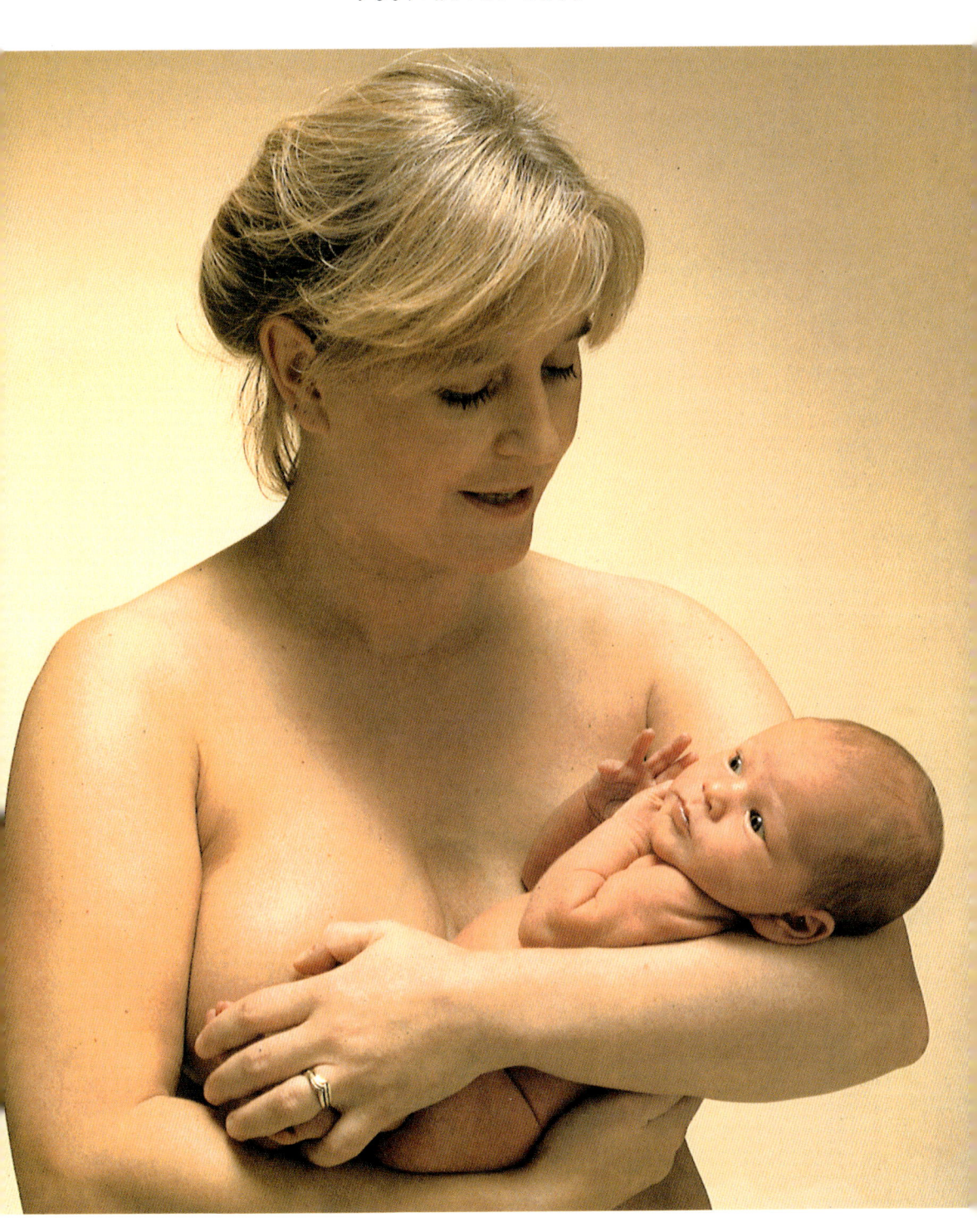

POST-NATAL CARE

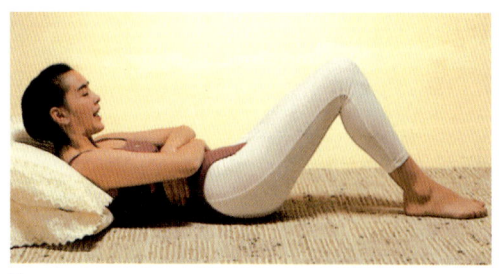

1 *Curl-ups: This exercise will help strengthen your vertical abdominal muscles. Lie on your back with a pillow under your head, your knees bent and your feet flat on the floor.*

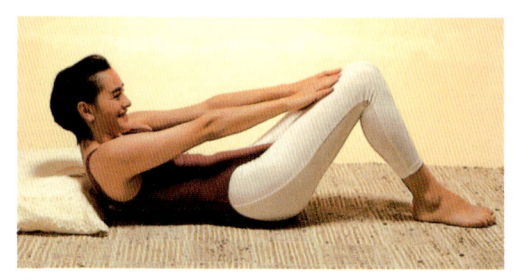

2 *Pull in your abdominal muscles and, raising your head, stretch your arms towards your knees. Hold for the count of five and then relax slowly. Repeat several times.*

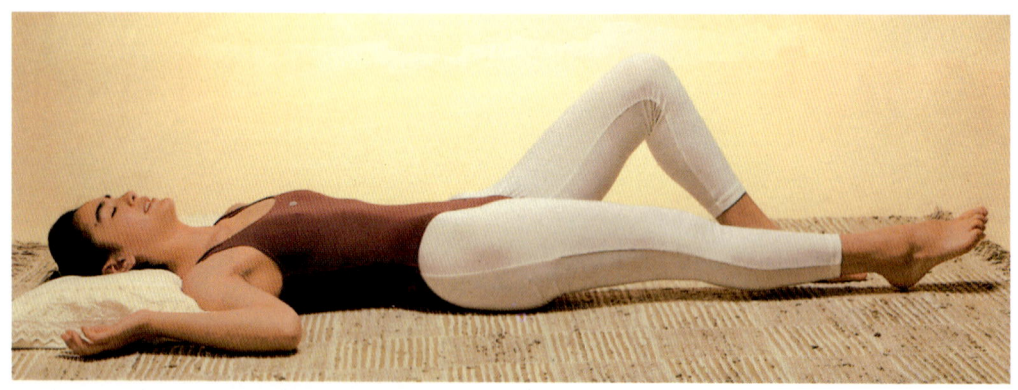

Leg slide: Lie with your head on a pillow with the small of your back pressed against the floor and your knees bent. Gently slide one leg away from your body until it is fully extended, keeping the small of your back pressed against the floor for as long as you can. Slowly draw the leg back towards your body and then repeat with the other leg. Do this several times.

return to its original size. If you are breast-feeding you may feel it contract as you feed the baby.

If your perineum (the skin between the vagina and anus) was bruised during labour, or if you had stitches, you will find that anything that puts pressure on the area painful. Soreness can be soothed with an ice pack (or ice cubes wrapped in a flannel) held against the perineum or by splashing with warm water. Try drying the area with a hand-held hair dryer, set on cool, rather than with a bath towel. Do not put the dryer too close to your skin, or use it in the bathroom. Adding a cup of salt to the bath water will also help the stitches to heal.

Getting back into shape

Despite losing the combined weight of the baby, the placenta, and the amniotic fluid, you will still be heavier than you were before you became pregnant. You may even find that you have to continue to wear maternity clothes for a short while. As your uterus shrinks during the six weeks following the birth you will lose more weight, but you will need to watch your diet to regain your pre-pregnancy shape. Try to eat regularly and healthily and don't be tempted, because you're short of time, to snack on foods containing empty calories such as sweets and fizzy drinks. If the weight isn't disappearing as fast as you'd like, ask your health visitor for advice. Do not attempt any diet now or while you are breast-feeding – this would simply increase stress as your body is struggling to regain its equilibrium. Doing exercises will help you get

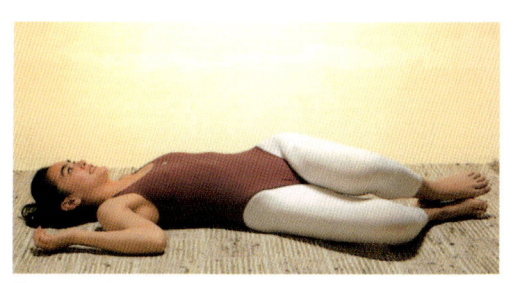

1 *Waist trimmer: Lie on the floor with your arms away from your side, with your knees bent and feet flat. Pull in your abdominals and, with knees together, roll over to the right. Take your knees back to the middle and pause.*

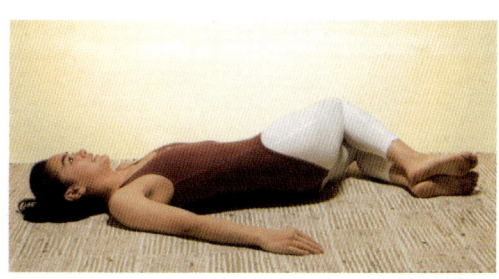

2 *Rest briefly, then pull in your abdominals again and roll your knees to the left, then back to the middle and pause. Keep your shoulders flat on the floor as you roll from side to side. Repeat six times and work up to 20.*

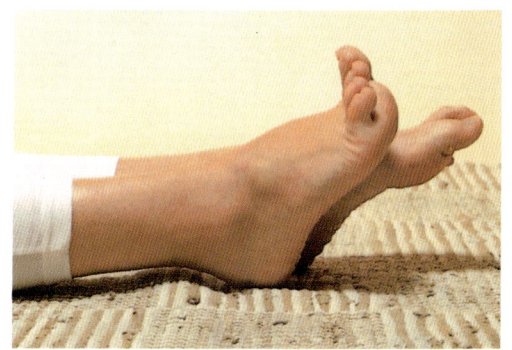

1 *Foot exercises: These will help improve your circulation and are especially important if you are confined to bed. Lie with your legs straight and knees together and bend and stretch your feet.*

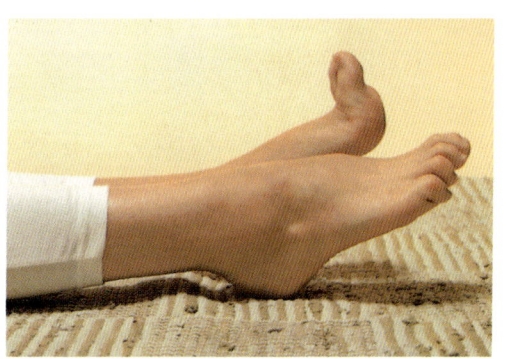

2 *Flex one foot, pulling the toes up towards you while pointing the other foot away from you. Repeat, alternating the feet. Do this exercise quite briskly for about 30 seconds.*

Post-natal depression

Two or three days after the birth you may suddenly feel very tearful and depressed. This is commonly called the "third day blues", or the milk blues, because it usually coincides with the milk coming into your breasts. These feelings are caused by all the hormonal changes that are going on in your body and should disappear after a few days. If they don't go away, however, you need to talk to your health visitor or doctor. You may be suffering from post-natal depression (PND) which, if left untreated, can go on for several months. Symptoms of PND include feeling unhappy and wretched as well as irritable and exhausted, yet unable to sleep. You may also lose all interest in food, or find yourself eating too much and then feeling guilty afterwards. PND is one of the most common illnesses following childbirth and it is likely that it is related to the huge hormonal changes that take place at the time of the birth, but it is still unclear as to why it affects some women so badly but not others. If you think you are suffering from PND, don't feel ashamed and don't ignore it. You need help and the sooner you ask for it the sooner you will begin to feel better and able to cope with life again. Post-natal depression is a common condition. Many women are affected by it, and it needs to be treated early on, not ignored in the hope that it will just go away on its own.

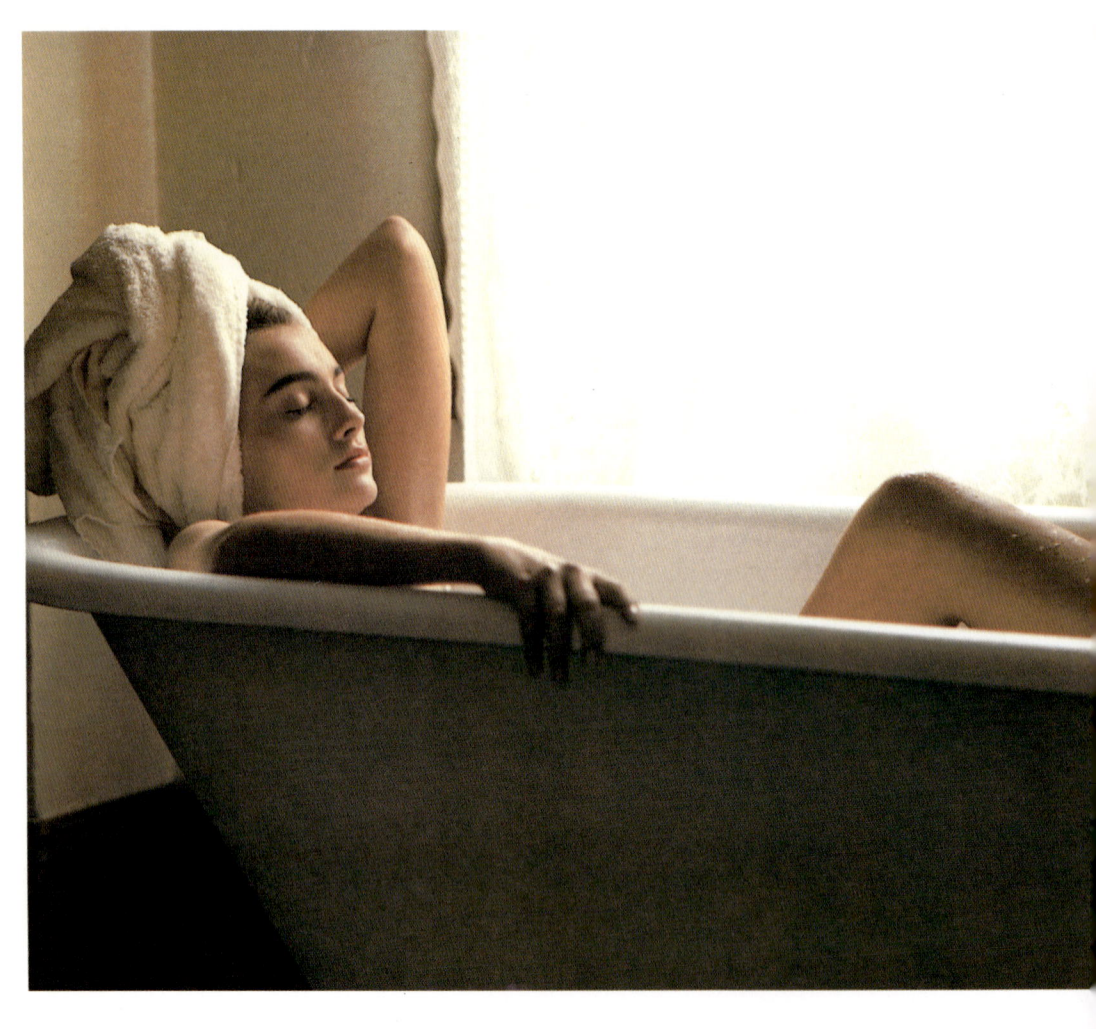

your figure back, get you moving again, and make you feel fitter. Those for strengthening the pelvic floor are among the most important post-natal exercises. The pelvic floor muscles support the bladder, uterus, and rectum, so it is vital that their tone is restored after being stretched during childbirth.

TIREDNESS AND RELAXATION
Tiredness goes hand in hand with being a new mother, but you need rest to help your body recover from childbirth. It is tempting to use the baby's sleep times to catch up on chores, but do try to have a nap or proper rest at least once during the day. You and your child are more important than housework, so find ways to cut down the work. Accept offers of help and, if no one volunteers, don't be afraid to ask people.

Another way to cope with tiredness or stress is relaxation, so try using the ante-natal relaxation exercises to help you now. Also a long, lazy bath with a few drops of relaxing oil in the water will work wonders. For a real treat, ask your partner to give you a massage using a specially formulated oil before you go to sleep.

HAIR AND NAILS
The condition of your hair is likely to change during this time. It may become more greasy, or the opposite may happen and it will become noticeably drier than before. You may also suffer an increase in hair loss or your hair may seem a lot thicker than it did before you

POST-NATAL CARE

became pregnant. Whichever condition applies to you, wash your hair using a mild shampoo and avoid rubbing or brushing oily hair too much as this will only stimulate the sebaceous glands to produce more oil. Dry hair should be conditioned after every wash and, if possible, allowed to dry naturally.

Your nails are made of the same tissue as your hair, so if you are having problems with one you are likely to have problems with the other. These are due to fluctuating hormone levels and as soon as these settle your hair and nails will return to normal. Meanwhile, include enough protein and B vitamins in your diet because these will help improve the condition of both your hair and nails.

Left: When bleeding has stopped, a lazy bath with a few drops of oil, such as lavender, will help you to relax.
Below: A stimulating rub with a loofah brush or mitt will help remove dead cells on the skin's surface, and will stimulate the circulation.
Below right: Try using some unscented soap or a soapless cleansing bar if your skin is very itchy.

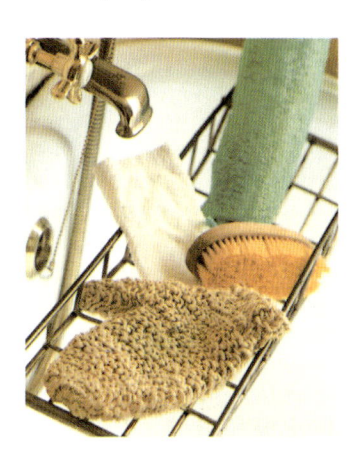

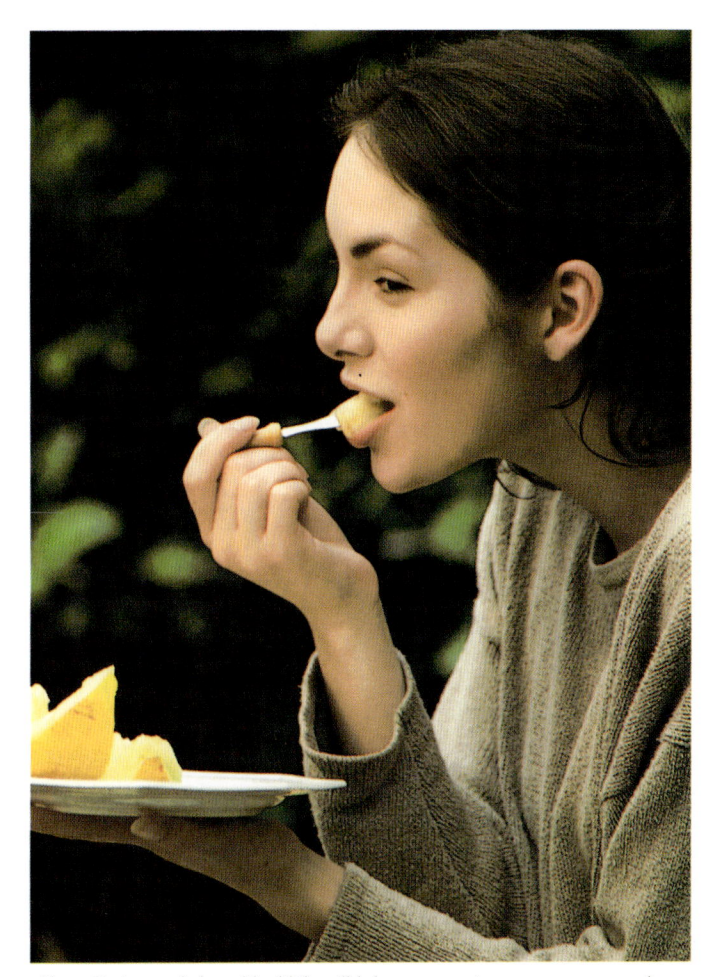

Above: Eating regularly and healthily will help you to regain your pre-pregnancy shape.

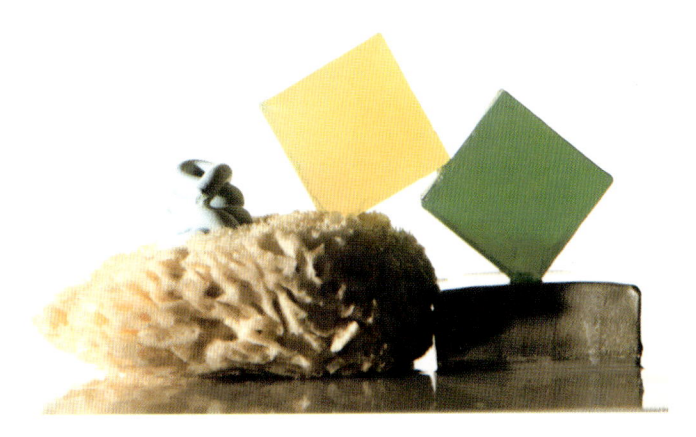

GLOSSARY OF PREGNANCY TERMS

ABORTION
The spontaneous or induced delivery of the fetus before the 28th week.

ABRUPTIO PLACENTAE
Part of the placenta peels away from the wall of the uterus in late pregnancy and often results in bleeding.

ALPHA-FETOPROTEIN (AFP)
A protein produced by the fetus which enters the mother's bloodstream. A very high level can indicate neural tube defects of the fetus such as Down's syndrome or spina bifida, but it can also mean that the woman is carrying more than one child.

AMNIOCENTESIS
A small amount of amniotic fluid is taken from the uterus through a needle inserted through the woman's abdomen and tested for chromosomal disorders such as Down's syndrome.

AMNIOTIC FLUID
The fluid surrounding the fetus in the uterus.

AMNIOTIC SAC
The bag of membranes which is filled with amniotic fluid in which the fetus floats during pregnancy.

ANAEMIA
A condition where the level of red corpuscles in the blood is abnormally low, which is treated with iron supplements.

ANALGESICS
Painkilling drugs which do not cause unconsciousness. The analgesics most commonly used during labour are Entonox (a mixture of nitrous oxide and oxygen, known as "gas and air"), pethidine and meptid.

ANTE-NATAL
Before birth.

APGAR SCORE
A simple test to assess the baby's condition after birth.

BEARING DOWN
The pushing movement made by the uterus during the second stage of labour.

BIRTH CANAL
See Vagina.

BLASTOCYST
The early stage of the developing embryo when it becomes a cluster of cells.

BRAXTON HICKS CONTRACTIONS
Contractions of the uterus which occur throughout pregnancy, but may not be felt until the last month or so. They feel like a painless, but sometimes uncomfortable, hardening across the stomach.

BREECH PRESENTATION
The position of a baby when he is bottom down rather than head down in the uterus.

CAESARIAN SECTION
Delivery of the baby through a cut in the abdomen and uterine walls.

CERVIX
The neck of the uterus or womb which is sealed with a plug of mucus during pregnancy. During labour, muscular contractions open up the cervix until it is about 10 cm/4 in wide so that the baby can pass through it into the vagina.

CHLOASMA
Slight discoloration of the skin, usually on the face, which occurs during pregnancy and disappears within weeks of the birth.

CHORIONIC VILLUS SAMPLING
A screening test for genetic handicap which can be done as early as 11 weeks. Cells are taken from the tissue that surrounds the fetus and are then analysed.

COLOSTRUM
A fluid that the breasts produce during pregnancy and immediately after the birth. It is full of nutrients and contains antibodies which will protect the baby from some infections.

CONCEPTION
The fertilization of the egg by the sperm and its implantation in the wall of the uterus.

CONGENITAL ABNORMALITIES
An abnormality or deformity that exists from birth. It is caused by a damaged gene or the effect of some diseases during pregnancy.

CONTRACTIONS
Regular tightening of the muscles of the uterus as they work to dilate the cervix and push the baby down the birth canal.

CROWNING
The moment when the crown of the baby's head appears in the vagina.

DILATION
The gradual opening of the cervix during labour.

DOPPLER
A method of using ultrasound vibrations to listen to the fetal heart.

ECTOPIC PREGNANCY
A pregnancy which develops outside the uterus, usually in the Fallopian tube.

EDD
Estimated date of delivery.

ELECTIVE INDUCTION
Induction done for convenience rather than for medical reasons.

ELECTRONIC FETAL MONITORING
The continuous monitoring of the fetal heart.

EMBRYO
The name of the developing organism in pregnancy from about the 10th day after fertilization until the 12th week of pregnancy when it becomes known as a fetus.

ENGAGED
The baby's head is engaged when it drops down deep in the pelvic cavity so that the widest part is through the mother's pelvic brim. Another term for this is "lightening". Most babies are born head first and will have engaged before labour begins.

ENGORGEMENT
The breasts become congested with milk if long periods are left between feeds which results in painful engorgement.

ENTONOX
Gas and oxygen, a short-term analgesic, which can be inhaled during labour.

EPIDURAL
An anaesthetic which is injected into the fluid surrounding the spinal cord at the base of the spine to relieve pain but leave the mother fully conscious.

EPISIOTOMY
A small cut made in the perineum to enlarge the vagina if there is a risk of tearing when the baby's head is about to be born.

FALLOPIAN TUBES
Two narrow tubes about 10 cm/4 in long which lead from the ovaries to the uterus.

FETUS
The developing baby from the end of the embryonic stage at about the 12th week of pregnancy, until the date of delivery.

FH
Fetal heart.

FMF
Fetal movement felt.

FOLIC ACID
A form of vitamin B which is important for the healthy development of the embryo. A daily supplement of 0.4mg should be taken before becoming pregnant and then until the 12th week of pregnancy.

FONTANELLES
The soft spots between the unjoined sections of the skull of the baby.

FORCEPS
An instrument sometimes used to assist the baby out of the birth canal.

FOREMILK
The first breast milk the baby gets when he begins to suck which satisfies his thirst before the hind milk comes through.

FUNDUS
The top of the uterus.

GAS AND AIR
See Entonox

Glossary of Pregnancy Terms

Genetic Counselling
Advice on the detection and risk of recurrence of inherited disorders.

Gestation
The length of time between conception and delivery (usually around 40 weeks).

GP Unit
A special unit, usually in a hospital, where a pregnant woman gives birth under the care of her GP and midwife.

Haemoglobin (Hb)
The pigment that gives blood its red colour and contains iron and stores oxygen.

Haemorrhage
Excessive bleeding.

Haemorrhoids (Piles)
A form of varicose veins around the anus.

Hindmilk
The calorie-rich breast milk that follows the foremilk during feed.

Hormone
A chemical produced by the body to stimulate organs within the body, particularly those to do with growth and reproduction,

Human Chorionic Gonadotrophin (HCG)
A hormone produced early in pregnancy by the developing placenta. Its presence in the urine is used to confirm pregnancy.

Implantation
The embedding of the fertilized egg in the wall of the uterus.

Incompetent cervix
A weakened cervix that is unable to hold the fetus in the uterus for the full nine months. Sometimes a cause of late miscarriage or premature birth.

Induction
The process of artificially starting off labour.

Intravenous Drip
The infusion of fluids directly into the bloodstream through a fine tube into a vein.

Jaundice
Neonatal jaundice often occurs in newborn babies because of the inability of the liver to successfully break down an excess of red blood cells.

Labour
The process of childbirth.

Lanugo
A very fine covering of hair which appears all over the fetus during late pregnancy.

Lie
The position of the fetus in the uterus.

Lightening
See Engaged.

Linea Nigra
A line of dark pigmentation which appears down the centre of the abdomen on some women during pregnancy.

Lochia
Post-natal vaginal discharge.

Meconium
The green matter passed from the baby's bowels during the first days after birth. Meconium in the amniotic fluid before delivery is usually a sign of fetal distress.

Miscarriage
The loss of a baby before 24 weeks gestation.

Monitor
Machine or instrument to measure the baby's heartbeat and breathing.

Moulding
The shaping of the bones of the baby's skull as it passes through the birth canal.

Mucus
A sticky secretion.

NAD
A medical term often used on medical records meaning "nothing abnormal detected".

Neural Tube Defect
Development defect of the brain and/or spinal cord.

Obstetrician
Medical specialist in pregnancy and childbirth.

Oedema
Swelling caused by fluid retention.

Ovary
Female organ responsible for production of sex hormones and eggs (ova).

Ovulation
The production of a ripe egg by the ovary, usually on a monthly basis.

Palpation
Manual examination of the uterus through the wall of the abdomen.

Pelvic Floor
The muscles which support the bladder and the uterus.

Perinatal
Period from before delivery until seven days after the birth.

Perineum
The area between the opening of the vagina and the anus.

Pethidine
A drug given during labour for pain relief and relaxation.

Placenta
Also known as "afterbirth", this is the fetus's life-support system which is attached to one side of the wall of the uterus and to the baby by means of the umbilical cord. All the fetus's nourishment passes from the mother through the placenta while the fetus's waste products pass out through it.

Premature or Preterm
A baby born before the 37th week.

Presentation
The position of the fetus in the uterus before and during the delivery.

Primigravida
A woman who is having her first baby.

Prostaglandin
A hormone which stimulates the onset of labour contractions.

Quickening
The first movements of the fetus in the uterus.

Rooting
The baby's instinctive searching for the mother's nipple.

Rubella (German Measles)
A virus which can be dangerous if caught during the first three months of pregnancy.

Scan
A way of screening the fetus in the uterus by bouncing high-frequency sound waves off it which build up a picture.

Shared Care
Ante-natal care shared between a GP and a hospital consultant.

Show
A vaginal discharge of blood-stained mucus that occurs before or during labour.

Stillbirth
The delivery of a baby who has already died in the uterus after 28 weeks of pregnancy.

Stretch Marks
Silvery lines that may appear where the skin has been stretched during pregnancy.

Term
The end of pregnancy - around 40 weeks from the date of conception.

Termination
An artificially induced abortion before the end of 28th week of pregnancy.

Toxoplasmosis
A parasitic disease spread by cat faeces that can cause blindness in a baby.

Trimester
Pregnancy is divided into three trimesters, each making up one third of pregnancy.

Umbilical Cord
The cord connecting the fetus to the placenta.

Uterus (Womb)
The hollow muscular organ in which the fertile egg becomes embedded.

Vacuum Extractor (Ventouse)
An instrument sometimes used to pull the baby out of the vagina.

Vagina
The birth canal through which the baby makes its way from the uterus.

INDEX

Page numbers in italic refer to the illustrations

abbreviations and terms, 23
abdomen, after delivery, 86
abdominal pain, 74
abortion, 92
abruptio placentae, 61, 92
aches and pains, 74
active birth, 54, *54*, 55, 56-7, *57*
acupuncture, 47, *79*
air travel, 62
alcohol, 8
alpha fetoprotein (AFP), 20, 92
amniocentesis, 20, *20*, 70, 92
amniotic fluid, 27, 82, 92
amniotic sac, 11, 92
anaemia, 45, 58, 60, 92
anaesthetics, 78, *79*
analgesics, 92
ante-natal care, 14-15, 18-21, 70, 92
ante-natal classes, 54-5, 68, *69*
Apgar score, 92
aromatherapy, 47, *47*, *79*
artificial rupture of the membranes (ARM), 78
asthma, 52

backache, 24, *47*, 62, *63*
bearing down, 92
bending in pregnancy, 62, *63*
birth *see* labour
birth canal, 92

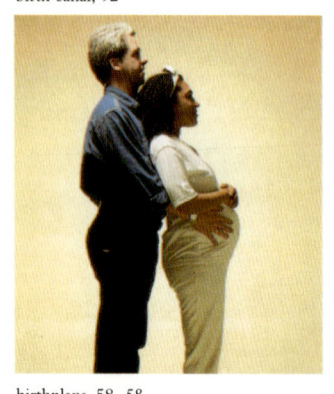

birthplans, 58, *58*
blankets, 51
blastocyst, 92
bleeding:
 in early pregnancy, 16
 in late pregnancy, 74
 placental problems, 60-1
blood pressure, 16, *16*, *17*, 18, 70
blood tests, 19, *19*, 20
bottle-feeding, 53, 86
bras:
 during pregnancy, 36, 42, *42*, 56, 64
 nursing bras, 52, 64
Braxton Hicks contractions, 30, 64-5, 80, 92
breast-feeding, 52-3, *52*, *53*, 86
breasts:
 bras, 36, 42, *42*, 52, 64

colostrum, 42, 58, 86
 during pregnancy, 52
 toning, *41*
breathing techniques, 55
breathlessness, 64, 76
breech birth, 80, *80*
breech presentation, 92
buggies, 50-1, *50-1*

Caesarean birth, 57, *85*
Caesarean section, 92
car seats, 51, *51*
car travel, 62, *62*
cervix, 92
cervical smear test, 86
cervix, dilation, 66, 82, 84
children, and new babies, 69
chloasma, 92
cholestasis, 44
chorionic villus sampling (CVS), 20-1, 92
chromosome disorders, 21, 70
clothes:
 baby's, 50-1, *50*
 during pregnancy, 36, *36-7*
colostrum, 42, 58, 86, 92
complications, during birth, 80-1
conception, 10-11, *10-11*, 92
congenital abnormalities, 92
constipation, 24
contraception, 8, 86
contractions: 92:
 Braxton Hicks, 30, 64-5, 80, 92
 breathing techniques, 55
 first stage of labour, 82, 83
 positions for labour, 66
 sexual intercourse and, 30, 31
cordocentesis, 21
cortisone, 76
cots, 51
cramp, 24
cravings, 42
crowning, 92
curl-ups, *88*
cystic fibrosis, 20

depression, post-natal, 89
diet:
 after delivery, 88
 during pregnancy, 26-7, *26-7*, 32, 33
 preparation for pregnancy, 9
 see also feeding
dilation, 92
discharges, vaginal, 25, 86
discomfort during pregnancy, 24-5, 64-5, 74-5
doctors, 14, 28-29, 86
doppler, 92
Domino scheme, 15
Down's syndrome, 20, 70
dreams, 68

ectopic pregnancy, 16-17, 92
eczema, 52
EDD, 92
egg (ovum), fertilization, 10, *11-12*
elective induction, 92
electronic fetal monitoring, 81, *81*, 92
embryo, 10, 92
emotions, in late pregnancy, 68-69
employment, during pregnancy, 32-3
engaged, 92

engagement, baby's head, 76
engorged breasts, 92
Entonox, 78, 92
epidural anaesthetic, 57, 78, *79*, 92
episiotomy, 57, 81, 84, 85, 92
equipment, baby's, 50-1, *50*
estimated date of delivery (EDD), 13, *13*, 82
exercise:
 during pregnancy, 40, *40-1*, 65
 post-natal exercises, 86, *86-9*, 89-90
 preparing for pregnancy, 9, *9*
expressing milk, 52-3

fainting, 24, 56
Fallopian tubes, 10, 16-17, 92
feeding:
 bottle-feeding, 53, 86
 breast-feeding, 52-3, *52*, *53*, 86
feet:
 exercises, *41*, *89*
 fluid retention, 16, 19, 38, 44-5, *45*
fertilization, 10, *10-11*
fetus, 92:
 abnormalities, 20-1, 70
 distress, 70
 engagement of head, 76
 kick charts, 65, *65*
 monitoring, 56, 70-1, 81, *81*
 movements, 44, 45
FH, 92
fluid retention, 16, 19, 38, 44-5, *45*
FMF, 92
folic acid, 9, 26, 92
fontanelles, 92
food cravings, 42
forceps delivery, 80, 92
foremilk, 92
formula milk, 53
fundus, 92
furniture, nursery, 49

gas and air, 78, *78*, 92
general practitioners (GPs), 28-29
genetic counselling, 21, *21*, 92
German measles (rubella), 8-9, 19, 86
gestation, 92
glue ear, 52
GP unit, 93
gums, bleeding, 20, 24, 36

haemoglobin, 93
haemorrhage, 93
haemorrhoids, 24-5, 93
hair:
 after pregnancy, 90-1
 during pregnancy, 38, *38*
head, engagement, 76
health hazards, 32-3
health visitors, 28, *29*
heartburn, 42, 44, *44*
height, mother's, 18-19
high blood pressure, 16
high chairs, *51*
high-tech birth, 57
home birth, 14-15, *85*
hormones, 93:
 during pregnancy, 22-3
 induction of labour, 78
 menstrual cycle, 10
 pregnancy tests, 12

INDEX

hospitals:
    final preparations, 72-3
    hospital birth, 15, *15*, 56, *56*
    parentcraft classes, 54
human chorionic gonadotrophin (HCG), 22, 93
hygiene, bottle-feeding, 53
hypnosis, 79

immunization, mothers, 8-9, 62, 86
implantation, 93
incompetent cervix, 93
induction of labour, 31, 57, 78, 93
injections, pain relief, 78
insomnia, 44, *44*
intensive care baby unit (ICBU), 76-7
internal examination, 19, 75, 86
intravenous drip, 93
iron, in diet, 58, 60
itching, 44

jaundice, 93

kick charts, 65, *65*
kidney infections, 60, 62

labour, 93:
    birthplans, 58, *58*
    choices in, 56-7
    complications, 80-1
    induction, 31, 57, 78
    older mothers, 70-1
    pain relief, 78-9, *79*
    positions, 66-7, *66-7*
    signs of, 82
    stages of, 83-4
lanugo, 35, 76, 93
leg slide exercise, *88*
lie, 93
"lightening", 76, 93
linea nigra, 93
listeria, 32
lochia, 88, 93

"mask of pregnancy", 38
massage, during pregnancy, 47, *47*, 79, 90
maternity record cards, 23
maternity rights and benefits, 36
mattresses, cot, 51
meconium, 93
medicines, 8
menstrual cycle, 10
meptid, 78
midwives, 14, 15, 28, 84
milk:
    bottle-feeding, 53
    breast-feeding, 52
miscarriage, 16, 17, 93
monitor, 93
monitoring, fetal, *56*, 70-1, 81, *81*
morning sickness, 13, 14
Moses baskets, *49*, 51
moulding, 93
mucus, 93

NAD, 93
nails, mother's, 42, *42*, 91
National Childbirth Trust (NCT), 55
natural birth, 56, *57*, 78
nausea, 13, 14, 74-6
nesting instinct, 77
neural tube defects, 9, 93
nipples, during pregnancy, 42, 52, *53*
nitrous oxide, 78, *78*
nursery, preparation, 48-9, *48-9*
nursing bras, 52, 64
nutrition, 9

obstetricians, *28*, 29, 93
oedema, 16, 19, 38, 44-5, *45,* 93
older mothers, 70-1
orgasm, 30
ovaries, 10, *10*, 49, 93
ovulation, 10, 93
oxygen, during labour, 55

pain, in late pregnancy, 74
pain relief, 57, 78-9, *79*
palpation, 93
parentcraft classes, 54-5, 68
partners:
    during birth, 58-9, *59*
    emotions, 68
pediatricians, 29, *29*
pelvic floor, 93
pelvis:
    during labour, 66-7
    exercises, *41, 88*, 92
    size of, 19, 75, 80
perinatal, 93
perineum, 93:
    episiotomy, 57, 81, 84, 85
    soreness, 90
pessaries, induction of labour, 78
pethidine, 78, 93
piles, 24-5
placenta, 93:
    delivery of, 77, 85
    development of, 10-11
    placenta praevia, 60
    placental insufficiency, 61
positions for labour, 66-7, *66-7*
post-natal care, 86-91
post-natal depression (PND), 89
prams, 50-1, *50*
pre-eclampsia, 16
premature or preterm, 93
pregnancy tests, 12, *13*
premature babies, 71, 76-7
preparation for pregnancy, 8-9
presentation, 93
primigravida, 93
prostaglandins, 31, 78, 93

quickening, 93

reflexology, 79
relaxation, 46-7, 92
reproductive system:
    female, *10*
    male, *11*
rest, 38, *60-1*, 90
rhesus factor, 20
ribs, during pregnancy, 46
rooting, 93
rubella (German measles), 8-9, 19, 86, 93

sanitary towels, 86
scans, ultrasound, 34, *34*, 60, *70-1,* 93
sciatica, *55*
seat belts, 62, *62*
sex of child, 11
sexual intercourse, 17, 30-1
shared care, 93
show, 82, 93
skin care, 38, *38-9*, 43, 91
sleep, 44, 90
smoking, 8
special care baby units (SCBU), 76-7, *76*
sperm, 10, *11*
spina bifida, 9, 20, 70
squatting:
    during labour, 66-7, *67*
    exercises, *41, 55*
stillbirth, 93

stitches, 86, 88
stretch marks, 36, 42, *43*, 93
stretching exercises, *55*
swimming, *65*
syntocinon, 78

tampons, 86
Taylor exercises, *41*
term, 93
termination, 93
terms and abbreviations, 93
tiredness, 45, 90
toxoplasmosis, 32-3, 93
transcutaneous electrical nerve stimulation (TENS), 78-9, *79*
transitional stage, 84
travel, during pregnancy, 62
trimesters, 11, 93
triple/double test, 20
tummy toning exercises, *41, 86*
twins, 34, *35*, 77

ultrasound scans, 34, *34*, 60, *70-1*
umbilical cord, 15, 84, 93
urine tests, 12, 18, 86
uterus, 93:
    after delivery, 86-7
    Braxton Hicks contractions, 64-5, 80
    placental problems, 60-1

vaccination *see* immunization
vacuum extraction, 80, 93
vagina, 93
vagina, discharges, 25, 86
varicose veins, 42
vegetarian diet, 26
veins, varicose, 42
ventouse, 80
vernix, 43, 69, 79

waist trimmer exercise, 89
water birth, 56, *84*
waters, breaking, 82, 83
weight:
    after delivery, 88
    during pregnancy, 18, *18*, 20, 26-7, 50, 56
womb *see* uterus
work, during pregnancy, 32-3

USEFUL ADDRESSES

There is no need to feel alone during pregnancy or in the months after the birth. The organizations mentioned below are happy to offer help and support to anyone who contacts them. Remember to enclose an SAE when writing to them.

Ante-natal and Birth
Active Birth Centre, Bickerton House, 25 Bickerton Road, London N19 5JT.
Tel: 0171-561 9006

Association for Improvements in the Maternity Services (AIMS), 40 Kingswood Avenue, London NW6 6LS.
Tel: 0181-960 5585

Association of Radical Midwives (ARM), 62 Greetby Hill, Ormskirk, Lancs. L39 2DT.
Tel: 01695-572776

BLISS (Information for parents of special-care babies), 17-21 Emerald Street, London WC1N 3QL.
Tel: 0171-831 9393

British Pregnancy Advisory Service (BPAS), Austy Manor, Wootton Wawen, Solihull, West Midlands B95 6BX.
Helpline: 01564-793225

Foresight (The Association for the Promotion of Conceptual Care), 28 The Paddock, Godalming, Surrey GU7 1XD.
Tel/fax: 01483-427839. Contact at least four months prior to planned conception.

Independent Midwives Association, Nightingale Cottage, Shamblehurst Lane, Botley, Hants. S032 2BY.
(No phone number, but please send A5 SAE for register of independent midwives)

Maternity Alliance, 15 Britannia Street, London WC1X 9JN.
Tel: 0171-837 1265 (Mon, Tues, Thurs, Fri 9am–1pm. Wed 2pm–5pm)

The Miscarriage Association, c/o Clayton Hospital, Northgate, Wakefield, W. Yorks. WF1 3JS.
Tel: 01924 200799 (answerphone out of office hours)

National Childbirth Trust (NCT), Alexandra House, Oldham Terrace, London W3 6NH.
Tel: 0181-992 8637

SAFTA (Support after termination for abnormality), 73-75 Charlotte Street, London W1P 1LB.
Tel: 0171-631 0285

Smokers' Quitline,
Tel: 0171-487 3000

Stillbirth and Neonatal Death Society (SANDS), 28 Portland Place, London W1N 4DE.
Tel: 0171-436 7940
Helpline: 0171-436 5881 (10am–5.30pm)

Toxoplasmosis Trust, 61-71 Collier Street, London N1 9BE.
Helpline: 0171-713 0599

Twins and Multiple Births Association (TAMBA), PO Box 30, Little Sutton, South Wirral L66 1TH.
Tel: 0151-348 0020 (Mon to Fri 9am–1pm)

WellBeing (Health Research Charity for Women and Babies), 27 Sussex Place, Regent's Park, London NW1 4SP.
Tel: 0171-262 5337

Family Links
Contact-a-Family, 170 Tottenham Court Road, London W1P OHA.
Tel: 0171-383 3555

Gingerbread, 49 Wellington Street, London WC2E 7BN.
Tel: 0171-240 0953

Meet a Mum Association, 14 Willis Road, Croydon, Surrey CR0 2XX.
Tel: 0181-665 0357. Also post-natal depression and general advice.
Helpline: 0181-656 7318.

National Childminding Association 8 Masons Hill, Bromley, Kent BR2 9EY.
Tel: 0181-464 6164

National Council for One Parent Families, 255 Kentish Town Road, London NW5 2LX.
Tel: 0171-267 1361

Working for Childcare, 77 Holloway Road, London N7 8JZ.
Tel: 0171-700 0281

For New Parents
Association of Breastfeeding Mothers, 26 Holmshaw Close, London SE26 4TH.
Tel: 0181-778 4769

Association for Post-Natal Illness, 25 Jerdan Place, London SW6 1BE.
Tel: 0171-386 0868 (answerphone out of office hours)

Cry-sis, BM Cry-sis, London WC1N 3XX (Counsellors available between 9am–11pm)
Tel: 0171-404 5011

La Leche League of Great Britain, PO Box BM 3424, London WC1N 3XX.
Tel: 0171-242 1278. Helps and supports women who wish to breast-feed. (24-hour counselling service)